O D L
OXFORD DIABETES LIBRARY

Diabetes ...
Pregnancy

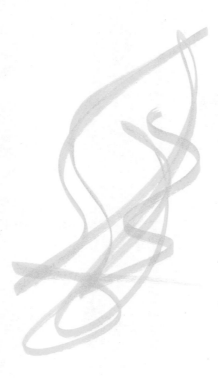

O D L
OXFORD DIABETES LIBRARY

Diabetes in Pregnancy

Edited by

Dr Robert Lindsay

Reader in Diabetes & Endocrinology,
British Heart Foundation Glasgow
Cardiovascular Research Centre,
University of Glasgow, UK

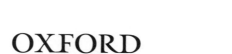

OXFORD
UNIVERSITY PRESS

OXFORD
UNIVERSITY PRESS

Great Clarendon Street, Oxford OX2 6DP,
United Kingdom

Oxford University Press is a department of the University of Oxford.
It furthers the University's objective of excellence in research, scholarship,
and education by publishing worldwide. Oxford is a registered trade mark of
Oxford University Press in the UK and in certain other countries

British Library Cataloguing in Publication Data

Data available

Library of Congress Cataloging in Publication Data

Data available

ISBN 978-0-19-959303-3

Printed in Great Britain by
Clays Ltd, St Ives plc

Contents

Preface

Diabetes in pregnancy encompasses a wide variety of problems in clinical management. Patients include those who may have had diabetes for many years, potentially with accompanying diabetes complications, and women newly diagnosed with gestational diabetes in that pregnancy. Clinical problems range from the need to tailor treatment regimens to the individual—for example to help a women with type 1 diabetes achieve near normal glycaemia—to the need in gestational diabetes to manage large scale programmes for the detection and treatment of diabetes in pregnancy.

From a public health perspective while the numbers of women with diabetes before pregnancy may be relatively small—perhaps 1 in 250 pregnancies in the UK—they have a disproportionately high number of complications in pregnancy. By contrast gestational diabetes is far more prevalent. The exact incidence in pregnancy will depend on the policies for screening and diagnostic criteria but it is likely that the incidence will range in most societies between 2 and 10% while adoption of the new international consensus on diagnosis may increase this to 16-20% of the population.

The field of diabetes in pregnancy is changing rapidly. For women with type 1 diabetes reports from a number of countries suggest that, while historically there have been huge improvements in rates of complications (particularly congenital malformation and perinatal mortality), these devastating complications remain stubbornly at two to three times the rate of the background population. Those managing type 1 diabetes have also had to consider use of the novel insulin analogues and insulin pump therapy (continuous subcutaneous insulin infusion (CSII)) as well as continuous glucose management systems.

Clinical developments are even greater in type 2 diabetes. First, in keeping with the epidemic of type 2 diabetes and obesity in the general population, there have been increases in the numbers of women with type 2 diabetes during pregnancy. Of greater concern as obesity in society increases and type 2 diabetes occurs at an earlier age the number of women with undiagnosed type 2 diabetes before pregnancy is also potentially increasing—a group at particular risk of poor control of diabetes in early pregnancy. The management of type 2 diabetes out of pregnancy has been developing rapidly—sulphonylureas and the biguanide metformin have been available for many years and thiazolidinediones for a little over 10 years. More recently drugs acting on the incretin axis such as the glucagon-like-peptide 1 (GLP-1) agonists and dipeptidyl peptidase IV (DPP-IV) inhibitors have been made available. Women may be on anti-obesity agents prior to their pregnancy while the use of cholesterol lowering medication—usually from the class of statins—has increased in this age group. While the newer agents for type 2 diabetes do not have a place in pregnancy management, they need to be considered in pre-pregnancy counselling. As the numbers of women with type 2 diabetes has increased it is has become appreciated that their pregnancy outcomes are usually equal or in some series worse than women with type 1 diabetes.

Finally, perhaps the most profound change has occurred in the management of gestational diabetes. The much-awaited Hyperglycaemia and Pregnancy Outcomes study was published in 2008, allowing an unprecedented window into the effects of normal and abnormal glucose tolerance on pregnancy outcomes. This is supplemented by two major randomized control trials examining the effect of diagnosis of gestational diabetes or "mild" gestational diabetes. These studies have for the first time conclusively shown the benefits of detection and treatment of gestational diabetes. Taken together these studies allow a rational reappraisal of how gestational diabetes is detected and diagnosed. Based on these and other studies, a new international consensus was reported in March of 2010 proposing new guidelines for screening and diagnosis of gestational diabetes. It is hoped that this will gain widespread international adoption as the various differences in screening and diagnosis have long slowed progress in the field. Treatment of gestational diabetes has also undergone important developments. Based on recent randomized control trials both glibenclamide and metformin have increased in acceptance—a timely development as the number of women with pregnancy complicated by diabetes has increased both due to underlying changes in obesity in the population and changing diagnostic criteria.

This short volume seeks to summarise some of these developments and bring together practical clinical advice on the management of diabetes in pregnancy. Longer volumes are available to give greater detail on the science behind some of these developments, and the aim here is to bring clinicians, nurses, and midwives up to date with some of the practical implications of the changes in this fast moving field.

Robert Lindsay

Abbreviations

AC	abdominal circumference
ACE	angiotensin-converting enzyme
ACEI	angiotensin-converting enzyme inhibitor
ACHOIS	Australian Carbohydrate Intolerance Study in Pregnant Women
ACR	albumin-to-creatinine ratios
ADA	American Diabetes Association
BGL	blood glucose level
CARDIA	Coronary Artery Risk Development in Young Adults
CGM	continuous glucose monitoring
CSII	continuous subcutaneous insulin infusion
CTG	cardiotocography
DCCT	Diabetes Control and Complications Trial
DM	diabetes
DPP	Diabetes Prevention Programme
FL	femur length
FPG	fasting plasma glucose
GDM	gestational diabetes mellitus
HAPO	Hyperglycaemia and Pregnancy Outcomes
HDL	high density lipoprotein
IADPSG	International Association of Diabetes And Pregnancy Study Groups
IDM	Infant of the Diabetic Mother
IGT	impaired glucose tolerance
IUGR	intrauterine growth restriction
LDL	low density lipoprotein
LMP	last menstrual period
MFMU	Maternal Fetal Medicines Unit Network
MODY	maturity onset diabetes of the young
NICE	National Institute for Health and Clinical Excellence
NPH	Neutral Protamine Hagedorn

OGCT	oral glucose challenge test
OGTT	oral glucose tolerance test
PGDM	pregestational diabetes
RCT	randomized controlled trial
RDS	Respiratory Distress Syndrome
SD	standard deviations
SIGN	Scottish Intercollegiate Guidelines Network
T1DM	type 1 diabetes
TRIPOD	TRoglitazone In Prevention Of Diabetes study
TTN	Transient Tachypnoea of the Newborn
WHO	World Health Organisation

Contributors

Dr Denice Feig
Head Diabetes and
Endocrinology in Pregnancy
Program
University of Toronto
Mount Sinai Hospital
60 Murray Street, Suite 5-027
Toronto
Ontario, Canada

Dr Lesley Jackson
Consultant Neonatologist/
Honorary Senior Lecturer
University of Glasgow,
Neonatal Unit,
Southern General Hospital,
Glasgow, UK

Dr Eleanor Jarvie
Clinical Research Fellow
Reproductive and Maternal
Medicine
University of Glasgow
Western Infirmary of Glasgow
Glasgow, UK

Dr Robert Lindsay
Reader in Diabetes &
Endocrinology
British Heart Foundation
Glasgow Cardiovascular
Research Centre,
University of Glasgow,
Glasgow, UK

Dr Helen R Murphy
Honorary Consultant/Senior
Research Associate
University of Cambridge
Metabolic Research
Laboratories
Institute of Metabolic Science
Cambridge, UK

Professor Scott M Nelson
Muirhead Chair in Obstetrics &
Gynaecology
Centre for Population and
Health Sciences
University of Glasgow
Glasgow, UK

Dr Rosemary Temple
Consultant in Diabetes and
Endocrinology,
Norfolk and Norwich
University Hospital NHS Trust
Norwich, UK

Chapter 1

Pre-pregnancy planning

Robert Lindsay

> **Key points**
>
> - Glycaemic control in early pregnancy bears a strong association with adverse pregnancy outcomes most notably congenital anomaly.
> - Pre-pregnancy planning is critical to allow optimization of medication and assessment of complications of diabetes.
> - Women should be advised of the risk of worsening of complications. If they have established nephropathy or macrovascular disease should only proceed to pregnancy if fully appraised of the potential ill effects on their or their child's health.
> - All women with diabetes should be encouraged to plan pregnancies and attend pre-pregnancy clinics.
> - Health professionals attending to women of childbearing age should raise women's awareness of the need for pre-pregnancy advice and planning.

1.1 Introduction

There is a strong relationship between the level of glycaemic control and a number of adverse outcomes in pregnancy. For this reason, along with the opportunity to prepare for pregnancy and ensure optimal maternal health before pregnancy, it is recommended that all women with diabetes plan pregnancies and attend for counselling before pregnancy to consider glycaemic control and other risk factors. There are numerous observational series which have demonstrated that women who attend pre-pregnancy counselling have lower maternal HbA$_{1c}$, lower rates of smoking and higher uptake of folic acid. While some of this difference will be accounted for by self-selection of women to pre-pregnancy counselling, services should be designed to try to encourage counselling before pregnancy. At a practical level there are a number of potential barriers to this. Pregnancy planning will require adequate access to contraceptive advice where desired. There may be barriers to pre-pregnancy advice based on ethnicity or social exclusion and services need to be responsive to this. An increasing issue in many countries is pre-pregnancy management of women with type 2 diabetes. In several countries women with type 2 diabetes of childbearing years may be more likely to be from ethnic minorities with potential language barriers to access to pre-pregnancy care. More generally women with type 2 diabetes may be more likely to be already treated with anti-hypertensive or cholesterol-lowering medication as well as oral or injected hypoglycaemic agents not suitable to pregnancy. Adequate pre-pregnancy counselling is all the more urgent in these women.

In this chapter we will consider evidence examining the relationship of maternal glycaemia to early pregnancy complications, issues relating to counselling women with complications of their diabetes as well as the broader role of pre-pregnancy counselling to improve health in during pregnancy.

1.2 Glycaemia in early pregnancy and pregnancy complications

A broad range of studies have demonstrated the relationship of maternal glycaemia to adverse outcomes in early pregnancy. The risk of congenital malformation is increased, as is the risk of miscarriage, as detailed in Figure 1.1. (Hanson et al., 1990). Guerin et al have summarized information from a number of sources giving

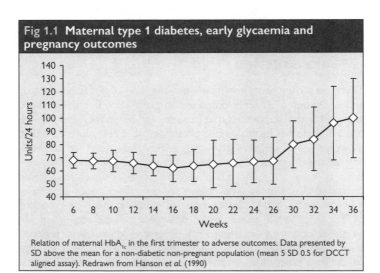

Fig 1.1 **Maternal type 1 diabetes, early glycaemia and pregnancy outcomes**

Relation of maternal HbA_{1c} in the first trimester to adverse outcomes. Data presented by SD above the mean for a non-diabetic non-pregnant population (mean 5 SD 0.5 for DCCT aligned assay). Redrawn from Hanson et al. (1990)

Table 1.1 Derived absolute risk of a major or minor congenital anomaly in association with the number of standard deviations (SD) of glycosylated haemoglobin above normal, and the approximate corresponding HbA$_{1c}$ concentration, measured periconceptionally

SD of GHb	Corresponding HbA$_{1c}$ (%)	Corresponding HbA$_{1c}$ (nmol/mol)	Absolute risk of a congenital anomaly (%, 95% CI)
0	5.0	31	2.2 (0.0 to 4.4)
2	6.0	42	3.2 (0.4 to 6.1)
4	7.0	53	4.8 (1.0 to 8.6)
6	8.0	64	7.0 (1.7 to 12.3)
8	9.0	75	10.1 (2.3 to 17.8)
10	10.0	86	14.4 (2.8 to 25.9)
≥12	≥11	≥97	20.1 (3. 0 to 37.1)

Assumes a DCCT-aligned HbA$_{1c}$ assay with mean (SD) of 5.0% (0.5%) among non-diabetic, non-pregnant controls. From Guerin A et al. (2007) Diabetes Care **30**: 1920–1925.

perhaps the best global estimate of the relationship of HbA$_{1c}$ to congenital malformation (Table 1.1) (Guerin et al., 2007). It should be noted that there is a steep relationship of first trimester HbA$_{1c}$ with risk of congenital malformation and it is recommended that this information is shared with women before pregnancy and support is given towards achieving optimal glycaemia.

The target level for HbA$_{1c}$ prior to withdrawal of contraception will differ between women. Guidelines vary as to the specific recommendations for level of glycaemic control prior to pregnancy. In 2008 NICE recommended that women should aim to maintain HbA$_{1c}$ under 6.1% (43 mmol/mol) if safely achievable (NICE, 2008). The Scottish Intercollegiate Guideline (2010) recommends that women should aim for an HbA$_{1c}$ of less than 7% (53 mmol/mol) although lower targets of HbA$_{1c}$ may be appropriate if maternal hypoglycaemia can still be minimized (Scottish Intercollegiate Guidelines Network, 2010). In most cases the limit to lowering glycaemia will be the risk of hypoglycaemia, severe hypoglycaemia and or hypoglycaemia unawareness. For this reason target HbA$_{1c}$ should be individualized.

For pre-pregnancy management where insulin injections are used, multiple dose regimens should be encouraged for all women allowing fine adjustment of dose in pregnancy. Selection of short and long-acting insulin regimens for pregnancy are discussed in Chapter 2 and will not be considered further here. In general women should be advised that insulin doses will increase through pregnancy. The absolute increase

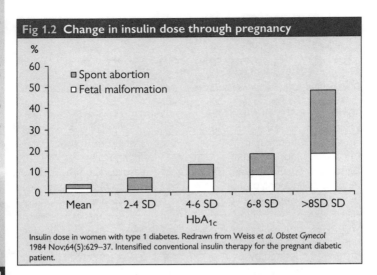

Fig 1.2 Change in insulin dose through pregnancy

- Spont abortion
- Fetal malformation

Insulin dose in women with type 1 diabetes. Redrawn from Weiss et al. *Obstet Gynecol* 1984 Nov;64(5):629–37. Intensified conventional insulin therapy for the pregnant diabetic patient.

varies but is of the order of an approximately 60% increase in most women with type 1 diabetes, with increases happening particularly after 18–20 weeks (Figure 1.2).

In most centres an attempt will be made to offer structured education to women before pregnancy. No randomized control trials of pre-pregnancy structured education exist but it would be expected that the improved HbA_{1c} and improved self-care and patient satisfaction seen in such programmes (DAFNE, 2002) would also translate into pre-pregnancy and such an approach is supported by guidelines (NICE, 2008; SIGN, 2010). Where glycaemic targets cannot be met without unacceptable levels of hypoglycaemia, consideration of continuous subcutaneous insulin infusion (CSII-insulin pump) is reasonable and again if this is likely to be necessary it is important that the change to CSII and necessary training and familiarization occurs before rather than during pregnancy, if possible. To date randomized control trials have not detected a systematic advantage of CSII in pregnancy (Mukhopadhyay et al., 2007) although it is recognized that these technologies are advancing rapidly and anecdotally advantages are seen, particularly in relation to nocturnal hypoglycaemia in individual cases.

For many women there is concern that hypoglycaemia and particularly severe hypoglycaemia may have a detrimental effect on their pregnancy. Evidence is limited. While severe induced hypoglycaemia does appear to be teratogenic in animal models (Buchanan et al., 1986) in general in human studies there has been no consistent association of maternal severe hypoglycaemia with congenital anomaly (Steel et al., 1990) or adverse developmental outcomes (Rizzo et al., 1991), and this observation is often reassuring to mothers. Nevertheless rigorous attempts need to be made to avoid hypoglycaemia and particularly severe hypoglycaemia.

1.3 Counselling women with diabetes complications

Complete assessment of complication prior to pregnancy and appropriate counselling is a key element of pre-pregnancy advice.

1.3.1 Diabetic nephropathy

Diabetic nephropathy is associated with an increased risk of deterioration of nephropathy and hypertensive disorders of pregnancy. Microalbuminuria is usually defined by albumin excretion of 20–200 µg/min or 30–300 mg/24 hours. These measures require timed or 24 hour collections of urine which can prove cumbersome and have been largely replaced by albumin-to-creatinine ratios (ACR) in two random or first morning urine specimens. ACR is highly correlated with longer measures in pregnancy (Justesen et al., 2006) and are much more straightforward for patients to supply. Microalbuminuria is generally defined by an ACR between 3.5–35 mg/mmol in women, although values as low as 2.5 mg/mmol may be considered abnormal in pregnancy due to higher creatinine clearance (Justesen et al., 2006). Albumin excretion levels greater than this (>300 mg/24 hours or ACR >35 mg/mmol) are in keeping with diabetic nephropathy.

There are a number of observational studies that have examined the rates of pregnancy complications in association with nephropathy. The study of Ekbom from 2001 in Denmark is summarized in Table 1.2. Notably there are very high rates of pre-eclampsia, low birth weight for gestational age, and pre-term delivery in association with both microalbuminuria and particularly in established nephropathy. A later, larger series from Denmark confirmed increases in pre-eclampsia (41%), and hypertension in the second trimester (13%) (Jensen et al., 2010). Microalbuminuria therefore appears to a have a particularly powerful association with pre-eclampsia and blood pressure in pregnancy. In the nephropathic group in the study of Ekbom the majority of women still had creatinine in the normal range (mean 91 µmol/l range 61–176 µmol/l). In a further series creatinine >130 µmol/l or proteinuria >3 g/24 hours were associated with delivery at gestational age 34 weeks on average and pre-eclampsia in 92% of cases (Gordon et al., 1996). Creatinine clearance increases by approximately 50% in normal pregnancy, and it is notable that in the small series available creatinine clearance often declines modestly in pregnancy complicated by diabetic nephropathy, while proteinuria may worsen particularly if baseline levels are >1 g/24 hours (Landon, 2007).

Aggressive treatment of risk factors may improve outcomes in pregnancy complicated by nephropathy. There are no large randomized control trials and we rely on reports from individual clinics where policies have adapted over time. Perhaps the best described of these again comes from the Danish series where control of blood pressure

Table 1.2 **Pregnancy complications in relation to microalbumin and nephropathy status**

	Normoalbu-minuria	microalbu-minuria	Nephropathy
n	166	26	11
Pre-term delivery before 37 weeks	35%	62%	91%
Pre-term delivery before 34 weeks	6%	23%	45%
Small for gestational age	2%	4%	45%
Pre-eclampsia	6%	42%	64%
Proteinuria >3 g/24 hours	0.5%	23%	55%
Jaundice requiring treatment	15%	8%	73%

Modified from Ekbom et al. (2001) Diabetes Care **24**: 1739–1744.

became tighter over time. A policy of introduction of antihypertensive agents to reduce blood pressure to targets of under 135/85, or introduction where urinary albumin excretion was > 0.3 g per 24 hours, was associated observationally with improved outcomes compared to historical controls from the same clinic (Nielsen et al., 2009). Notably however rates of pre-eclampsia in women with nephropathy were still 43%, and pre-term delivery (before 37 weeks) 71% although the total numbers were small (7 cases).

Taken together women should be counselled on the potential for blood pressure complications where microalbuminuria is present and counselled regarding the potential for more severe complications where overt nephropathy is present.

Finally, the longer term outlook for most women appears good. While anecdotally some women with established nephropathy experience a marked deterioration in renal function, on average women with microalbuminuria appear to suffer from no long-term decline in renal function as a result of pregnancy (DCCT 2000; Verier-Mine et al., 2005).

1.3.2 **Diabetic retinopathy**

Retinopathy may also deteriorate in pregnancy. This appears to be highly dependent on the grade of retinopathy present at the beginning of pregnancy. Thus while little deterioration is usually seen in women with no or minimal background retinopathy, up to 65% of women with frank retinopathy may progress (Laatikainen et al., 1980). Results from the DCCT (2000) demonstrate independent effects of both pregnancy and short term rapid improvements of glycaemic control to be associated with deterioration of retinopathy. Early pregnancy is often a time when glycaemic control improves rapidly and this offers another strong argument for pregnancy planning and pre-pregnancy counselling. In women with established retinopathy glycaemic control should be improved gradually pre-pregnancy to minimize the risk of progression.

In contemporary series up to 27% of women are found to have deterioration of retinopathy with 6% having sight-threatening change (Vestgaard et al., 2010). Sight-threatening progression was associated with diabetic macular oedema in early pregnancy, impaired visual acuity in early pregnancy and higher blood pressure throughout pregnancy (Vestgaard et al., 2010). All women should have retinal screening pre-pregnancy and at least three times during pregnancy to detect such progression. It is important to note that much of this disease will come under control with appropriate ophthalmological assessment and if necessary laser therapy. Counselling of women with established severe retinopathy is more complex.

In a similar fashion to nephropathy the longer-term outlook for the majority of patients appears to be good. Changes in retinopathy are often observed to regress after pregnancy. Across the lifespan pregnancy does not appear to be a risk factor for retinopathy, supporting the contention that changes during pregnancy are generally temporary (DCCT 2000; Verier-Mine et al., 2005). An exception to this is the presence of more severe degrees of retinopathy. When sight-threatening retinopathy is present in pregnancy, and laser therapy has been needed, retinopathy should not be expected to regress and further treatment postpartum is frequently needed (Chan et al., 2004).

1.3.3 **Diabetic neuropathy**

There are few reports of deterioration of either peripheral or autonomic neuropathy in pregnancy. In small studies there is no deterioration of nerve conduction simply in response to pregnancy (Lapolla et al., 1998). Pregnancy per se does not appear to be associated with any long-term deterioration in neuropathy (Verier-Mine et al., 2005). The presence of autonomic neuropathy and particularly diabetic gastroparesis is however of importance to pre-pregnancy counselling. These complications are often associated with difficulty in achieving excellent glycaemic control and with increased rates of hypoglycaemia. Gastroparesis is frequently associated with swings of blood sugar and difficulty in avoiding hypoglycaemia. An anecdotal literature suggests that gastroparesis is associated with maternal morbidity and even mortality in association with worsened problems of nausea and vomiting. Thus while the complications themselves may not be expected to worsen, careful thought should be taken over how tightly blood sugar will be able to be controlled and the difficulties that women will experience in pregnancy when neuropathy is present.

1.3.4 **Macrovascular disease**

Type 1 diabetes increases the risk of macrovascular disease. Relative risk of myocardial infarction and stroke mortality are increased dramatically in women with type 1 diabetes of childbearing years—by 40 fold and 7.6 fold respectively (Laing et al., 2003a; Laing et al., 2003b), although the absolute rates of these complications remain low (mortality from myocardial infarction women aged 20–29 13 per 100,000 person-years; women aged 30–39 82 per 100,000 person-years; stroke mortality aged 20–39 13 per 100,000 person-years) (Laing et al., 2003a; Laing et al., 2003b).

The presence of pre-existing macrovascular disease is a major concern in pregnancy. As women tend to deliver at older ages the frequency of pregnancy with pre-existing heart disease will be expected to increase. Pregnancy increases the risk of acute myocardial infarction 3–4 fold (Roth & Elkayam, 2008) and myocardial infarction in pregnancy carries a high maternal and fetal mortality (Roth & Elkayam, 2008). Most series are small and observational with no randomized evidence in this group. It is suggested that around 11% of women with acute myocardial infarctions in pregnancy have diabetes (Roth & Elkayam, 2008). Maternal mortality is 11% and fetal mortality 9%. These rates of mortality, although high, show an improvement compared to historical series but there would still appear to be a high rate of complications (Smith et al., 2008).

Such women with pre-existing vascular disease should be informed pre-pregnancy of these potential risks and may opt not to proceed to pregnancy. A multidisciplinary approach to counselling and management is advised.

1.4 **Pre-pregnancy counselling of women with hypertension and hypercholesterolaemia** (Table 1.3)

Women receiving antihypertensive and cholesterol lowering therapy before pregnancy require careful counselling. Many antihypertensives are contraindicated. Notably drugs interfering with the renin angiotensin system—the angiotensin converting enzyme inhibitors and angiotensin 2 receptor blocking agents—are considered nephrotoxic in the second and third trimesters. Exposure at this stage of pregnancy is associated with ACE-inhibitor fetopathy, a group

Table 1.3 Key points in pre-pregnancy counselling

- Assess glycaemic control (Hba_{1c} below 7% and if possible into the reference range)
- Assess complications of diabetes and counsel regarding the potential effects of pre-existing complications in pregnancy
- Encourage women to stop smoking
- Encourage folic acid
- Rubella testing
- Consider whether all medications will be compatible with pregnancy particular considerations to statins and ACE inhibitors.

of conditions that includes oligohydramnios intrauterine growth and abnormal renal development. More recently there has been more limited evidence of teratogenic effects of the ACEI in early pregnancy (Cooper et al., 2006). Exposure to ACEI in early pregnancy was associated with an almost three-fold increase in congenital anomalies (Cooper et al., 2006). For this reason women should be assessed pre-pregnancy and antihypertensives changed to agents generally considered safe in pregnancy. Recent guidance for more general use of antihypertensives during pregnancy suggests that labetalol, nifedipine and methyldopa are appropriate agents for use in pregnancy with labetalol being the first-line agent (NICE, 2010).

Clinical difficulty may arise in women attending for pre-pregnancy counselling who are already treated with multiple agents for blood pressure, particularly in the presence of nephropathy and heavy proteinuria. There is an anecdotal literature supporting continuation of ACEI up until conception, to attempt to maintain the benefits of these agents for as long as possible pre-pregnancy (Bar et al., 1999). This policy needs to be balanced against potential teratogenic effects and carefully discussed pre-pregnancy.

Similarly, an increasing number of women are exposed to cholesterol-lowering medication. There are reports of fetal limb anomalies and holoprosencephaly in association with exposure to statins in the first trimester (Edison & Muenke, 2004). Women should be counselled and the agents avoided.

1.5 Other factors

There is a general recommendation that higher doses of folic acid are used—4 or 5 mg rather than the usual level of 400 µg found in usual pregnancy multivitamins. Folic acid is of proven benefit in reducing the incidence of spinal cord abnormalities in pregnancy. It would not be expected to rescue other congenital anomalies.

There is a rich literature examining other agents in some animal models, with antioxidant vitamins being of particular interest in reducing anomalies. This has not yet been convincingly translated into the human situation. Pre-pregnancy advice should also cover the range of more general pre-pregnancy counselling. Women should be advised to stop smoking and offered support to do so. Pre-pregnancy testing for rubella is also appropriate.

1.6 **Conclusions**

It is clearly desirable for women to enter pregnancy understanding all of the potential complications. It is stressed that, with care and attention and appropriate support, outcomes are good for the majority of women—the potential exceptions being women with advanced degrees of nephropathy, retinopathy or macrovascular disease. Care should be taken to stress that many of the adverse outcomes can be avoided in the majority of cases and that an unduly negative picture is not given—this balance requires experience in counselling from teams seeing the broad range of women in pregnancy.

Further reading

Bar J, Chen R, Schoenfeld A, Orvieto R, Yahav J, Ben-Rafael Z, Hod M (1999). Pregnancy outcome in patients with insulin dependent diabetes mellitus and diabetic nephropathy treated with ACE inhibitors before pregnancy. *J Pediatr Endocrinol Metab* **12**: 659–65.

Buchanan TA, Schemmer JK, Freinkel N (1986). Embryotoxic effects of brief maternal insulin-hypoglycemia during organogenesis in the rat. *J Clin Invest* **78**: 643–9.

Chan WC, Lim LT, Quinn MJ, Knox FA, McCance D, Best RM (2004). Management and outcome of sight-threatening diabetic retinopathy in pregnancy. *Eye (Lond)* **18**: 826–32.

Cooper WO, Hernandez-Diaz S, Arbogast PG, et al. (2006). Major congenital malformations after first-trimester exposure to ACE inhibitors. *N Engl J Med* **354**: 2443–51.

DAFNE Study Group (2002). Training in flexible, intensive insulin management to enable dietary freedom in people with type 1 diabetes: dose adjustment for normal eating (DAFNE) randomised controlled trial. *BMJ* **325**: 746.

Diabetes Control and Complications Trial Research Group (2000). Effect of pregnancy on microvascular complications in the diabetes control and complications trial. *Diabetes Care* **23**: 1084–91.

Edison RJ, Muenke M (2004). Central nervous system and limb anomalies in case reports of first-trimester statin exposure. *N Engl J Med* **350**: 1579–82.

Gordon M, Landon MB, Samuels P, Hissrich S, Gabbe SG (1996). Perinatal outcome and long-term follow-up associated with modern management of diabetic nephropathy. *Obstet Gynecol* **87**: 401–9.

Guerin A, Nisenbaum R, Ray JG (2007). Use of maternal GHb concentration to estimate the risk of congenital anomalies in the offspring of women with prepregnancy diabetes. *Diabetes Care* **30**: 1920–5.

Hanson U, Persson B, Thunell S (1990). Relationship between haemoglobin A1C in early type 1 (insulin-dependent) diabetic pregnancy and the occurrence of spontaneous abortion and fetal malformation in Sweden. *Diabetologia* **33**: 100–4.

Jensen DM, Damm P, Ovesen P, et al. (2010). Microalbuminuria, preeclampsia, and preterm delivery in pregnant women with type 1 diabetes: results from a nationwide Danish study. *Diabetes Care* **33**: 90–4.

Justesen TI, Petersen JL, Ekbom P, Damm P, Mathiesen ER (2006). Albumintocreatinine ratio in random urine samples might replace 24-h urine collections in screening for micro- and macroalbuminuria in pregnant woman with type 1 diabetes. *Diabetes Care* **29**: 924–5.

Laatikainen L, Larinkari J, Teramo K, Raivio KO (1980). Occurrence and prognostic significance of retinopathy in diabetic pregnancy. *Metab Pediatr Ophthalmol* **4**: 191–5.

Laing SP, Swerdlow AJ, Carpenter LM, et al. (2003a). Mortality from cerebrovascular disease in a cohort of 23 000 patients with insulin-treated diabetes. *Stroke* **34**: 418–21.

Laing SP, Swerdlow AJ, Slater SD, et al. (2003b). Mortality from heart disease in a cohort of 23,000 patients with insulin-treated diabetes. *Diabetologia* **46**: 760–5.

Landon MB (2007). Diabetic nephropathy and pregnancy. *Clin Obstet Gynecol* **50**: 998–1006.

Lapolla A, Cardone C, Negrin P, et al. (1998). Pregnancy does not induce or worsen retinal and peripheral nerve dysfunction in insulin-dependent diabetic women. *J Diabetes Complications* **12**: 74–80.

Mukhopadhyay A, Farrell T, Fraser RB, Ola B (2007). Continuous subcutaneous insulin infusion vs intensive conventional insulin therapy in pregnant diabetic women: a systematic review and metaanalysis of randomized, controlled trials. *Am J Obstet Gynecol* **197**: 447–56.

National Institute for Health and Clinical Excellence (NICE) (2008). Diabetes in pregnancy. *Management of diabetes and its complications from preconception to the postnatal period. NICE clinical guideline*, 63. NICE, London.

National Institute for Health and Clinical Excellence (NICE) (2010). Hypertension in pregnancy: the management of hypertensive disorders during pregnancy (CG 107). NICE, London. http://www.nice.org.uk/nicemedia/live/13098/50418/50478.pdf

Nielsen LR, Damm P, Mathiesen ER (2009). Improved pregnancy outcome in type 1 diabetic women with microalbuminuria or diabetic nephropathy: effect of intensified antihypertensive therapy? *Diabetes Care* **32**: 38–44.

Rizzo T, Metzger BE, Burns WJ, Burns K (1991). Correlations between antepartum maternal metabolism and child intelligence. *N Engl J Med* **325**: 911–6.

Roth A, Elkayam U (2008). Acute myocardial infarction associated with pregnancy. *J Am Coll Cardiol* **52**: 171–80.

Scottish Intercollegiate Guidelines Network (2010). *Management of diabetes, a national clinical guideline*, 116. SIGN, Edinburgh.

Smith RL, Young SJ, Greer IA (2008). The parturient with coronary heart disease. *Int J Obstet Anesth* **17**: 46–52.

Steel JM, Johnstone FD, Hepburn DA, Smith AF (1990). Can prepregnancy care of diabetic women reduce the risk of abnormal babies? *BMJ* **301**: 1070–4.

Verier-Mine O, Chaturvedi N, Webb D, Fuller JH (2005). Is pregnancy a risk factor for microvascular complications? The EURODIAB Prospective Complications Study. *Diabet Med* **22**: 1503–9.

Vestgaard M, Ringholm L, Laugesen CS, Rasmussen KL, Damm P, Mathiesen ER (2010). Pregnancy-induced sight-threatening diabetic retinopathy in women with Type 1 diabetes. *Diabet Med* **27**: 431–5.

Chapter 2

Pregestational (type 1 and type 2) diabetes: care and complications during pregnancy

Helen R Murphy

Key points

- Fetal growth acceleration resulting in the delivery of a large for gestational age or macrosomic infant is the commonest complication of pregnancy affecting approximately 50% of diabetic pregnancies
- Macrosomic infants are at increased risk both of immediate birth complications (shoulder dystocia, neonatal hypoglycaemia and neonatal care admission) and of longer term complications (insulin resistance, obesity and type 2 diabetes)
- Pre-eclampsia complicates 13% or 1 in 7 diabetes pregnancies and is closely related to glycaemic control during the second trimester
- Quick acting analogues (NovoRapid® and Humalog®) are the preferred prandial insulins. Basal insulin replacement is controversial with NICE recommending only Neutral Protamine Hagedorn (NPH) or pump therapy during pregnancy.

13

2.1 Antenatal care of women with pregestational diabetes

2.1.1 Prevalence of type 1 and type 2 diabetes during pregnancy

Pregestational diabetes is the commonest medical complication of pregnancy, currently affecting approximately one in 250 pregnancies. The prevalence of diabetes in pregnancy is set to further increase, with a doubling in the incidence of type 1 diabetes in adolescents under the age of 15 years during the past two decades. As the obesity epidemic continues, the proportion of pregnancies complicated by type 2 diabetes is also increasing, with rapid rises across the UK during the past 5 years, such that 40% of diabetic pregnancies are now complicated by type 2 diabetes. The impact of these changes on maternity service provision cannot be underestimated as 90% women with type 2 diabetes are overweight or obese. These women are also older, of higher parity and more likely to have hypertension, cardiac disease and take potentially teratogenic medications (ACE inhibitors, statins). Half the women with type 2 diabetes belong to an ethnic minority group (predominantly Asian) and 45% live in a deprived area. The association of poor pregnancy outcome with maternal deprivation is particularly concerning, with over one third of stillbirths and neonatal deaths occurring in women from deprived areas.

2.1.2 Glycaemic control

Despite clear evidence that women who attend pre-pregnancy care have improved blood glucose control and reduced risk of congenital malformation, only 50% of diabetic pregnancies are planned and less than a third of women with diabetes receive adequate pre-conception care. Therefore a majority of women are poorly prepared for pregnancy and will be striving to achieve optimal glycaemic control during early pregnancy. At the booking visit, we focus on providing women and their partners with an honestly optimistic outlook regarding the risk of complications of pregnancy (Tables 2.1 and 2.2). We explain the physiological changes of pregnancy and describe our rationale for the risks and benefits of tight glycaemic control throughout pregnancy, focusing on strategies to manage:

- Glucose excursions/variability during pregnancy (before 6 weeks of gestation)
- Reduced hypoglycaemia awareness/risk of severe hypoglycaemia (6–16 weeks)
- Tight postprandial control to reduce pre-eclampsia/macrosomia (>16 weeks).

Table 2.1 Booking visit

- Document 1st day of last menstrual period (LMP) and contraception use during 12 months before pregnancy
- Screen for diabetic complications (retinal photography and urinary ACR)
- Document co-existing illnesses and medication use at conception
- Discontinue statins, ACE inhibitors and review the use of anticonvulsants (especially valproate) with neurology team
- High-dose 5 mg folic acid supplementation to be commenced and/or continued until dating scan confirms gestational age of 12 weeks
- Document smoking status and refer as appropriate for smoking cessation
- Document maternal height, weight and BMI and refer for Dietitian input
- Discuss risks of hypoglycaemia/loss of hypoglycaemic awareness during pregnancy with women and partners. Document driving advice and prescription of glucagon kit
- Review sick day rules and risk of ketoacidosis during pregnancy. Prescribe ketone testing equipment (Ketostix® or ketone testing strips)
- Provide support and encouragement for women to monitor their blood glucose levels regularly before and 1-hr after meals and before bed
- Negotiate targets for blood glucose levels and HbA$_{1c}$ advising that NICE recommend a fasting BGL 3.5–5.9 mmol/l and <7.8 mmol/l 1 hour after meals
- Review insulin:carbohydrate ratios and correction doses describing the likely changes (reduction in early pregnancy and potential large increases thereafter)
- Provide an honestly optimistic account of the pregnancy risks associated with diabetes:
  - Congenital malformation, stillbirth and neonatal death (3–5 times general maternity population) but >90% pregnancies have good outcome
  - Severe hypoglycaemia in 40% of pregnancies and although rare is leading cause of maternal death, but potentially preventable by frequent BG monitoring and support from partner, family, work colleagues etc
  - Pre-eclampsia 13% but can be reduced by tight glucose control in second trimester
  - Macrosomia 50% but can be reduced by tight post-prandial glucose control throughout the second and third trimesters
  - Induction of labour at 38 weeks gestation
  - Caesarean section 60% (but 30% elective and most "emergency" caesarean sections are due to failed induction)
  - Premature delivery <37 weeks (33%) but risks of earlier premature deliver <34 weeks can be reduced by tight glucose control
  - Neonatal care admission (33%) although commonly for neonatal hypoglycaemia which can be reduced by tight glucose control in labour and during late pregnancy.

2.1.3 **Dietary advice**

All women are offered individual dietary advice with review of their insulin:carbohydrate ratio, insulin sensitivity factors and approaches to correcting hypo- and hyperglycaemic excursions. Women who have not had structured education before pregnancy will be fast-tracked onto the next available course, whenever possible. For women who cannot attend structured education, pragmatic correction factors are suggested starting with 1 unit of quick-acting insulin to lower BGL by 2–3 mmol/l, and 1 unit of quick-acting insulin to cover 10g carbohydrate. We suggest that carbohydrate loads >60g are avoided and that more highly processed high glycaemic index foods with refined carbohydrate be replaced by low glycaemic index alternatives, e.g. granary bread instead of white or wholemeal, basmati rice instead of jasmine, and wholemeal instead of white pasta. It is important to remind women that insulin reduces endogenous or hepatic glucose production and increases glucose uptake into muscle, but does not directly influence the gut absorption of glucose, which is entirely dependent of the type and quantity of carbohydrate consumed. Hence the dietary freedom approaches to self management outside of pregnancy are less applicable when striving for very tight postprandial glucose control.

Women whose pre-pregnancy body mass index is >27 kg/m^2 (approximately 50% of women with type 1 diabetes and 90% with type 2 diabetes) are advised to restrict calorie intake (to 25 kcal/kg/day or less) as per the NICE recommendations for gestational diabetes. All women, regardless of their baseline body mass index, are advised to take moderate exercise of at least 30 minutes daily.

2.1.4 **Severe hypoglycaemia**
The proportion of women affected by severe hypoglycaemia during early pregnancy rises from 25% in the 12 months before pregnancy to 40% during the late first and early second trimester. This is important, as severe hypoglycaemia is the leading cause of maternal death in type 1 diabetes. Most women have reduced hypoglycaemic awareness between 8–16 weeks' gestation, with a lowering of the blood glucose level at which warning symptoms are first detected and either partial or complete loss of hypoglycaemic awareness. The most important risk factors include a past history of severe hypoglycaemia, long duration type 1 diabetes (>10 years), reduced hypoglycaemic awareness, tight glycaemic control (HbA$_{1c}$ <6.5%) and higher total daily doses of insulin (Farrar et al., 2007). Continuous subcutaneous insulin infusion (CSII) is the only intervention proven to reduce risk of severe hypoglycaemic during early pregnancy and should be offered to women at risk, arguably all women with longer duration type 1 diabetes.

We suggest that women inform their partner, family members and when applicable work colleagues regarding the risk of hypoglycaemia. We document and discuss the precautions required for driving (frequent BG testing and lack of severe hypoglycaemia) at every visit and advise that women with severe hypoglycaemia avoid driving until later in the second trimester, usually after 16–18 weeks. We advise women with or at increased risk of severe hypoglycaemia to avoid sleeping alone, if possible, particularly during early pregnancy. We are increasingly using real time continuous glucose monitoring devices with nocturnal alarms set for glucose threshold <4mmol/l in high risk women, with funding obtained on a named patient basis, when clinically indicated.

2.1.5 Daily hypoglycaemia

Milder episodes of maternal hypoglycaemia also cause significant maternal morbidity and are a major barrier to achieving tight glycaemic control during pregnancy. Using continuous glucose monitoring (CGM) we have shown that women with type 1 diabetes have on average 2.3 episodes of hypoglycaemia/24hr, spending approximately 3 hours with glucose levels <3.5 mmol/l (Hovorka, 2006). The proportion of time spent hypoglycaemic remained quite constant throughout pregnancy, suggesting that even after the risk of severe hypoglycaemia has reduced, diurnal and nocturnal hypoglycaemia persist. Although women with type 2 diabetes have fewer overall episodes of hypoglycaemia, on average 1.8 episodes lasting approximately 2 hours per day, their risk of nocturnal hypoglycaemia is equivalent to women with type 1 diabetes. They have often less experience dealing with hypoglycaemia before pregnancy and may require considerable reassurance and support to balance the benefits of tight control with risks of hyperglycaemia.

2.2 Insulin regimens during pregnancy

2.2.1 Prandial insulin

Insulin aspart (NovoRapid®) is the only commonly used analogue insulin with marketing authorization specific to pregnancy, and it is recommended that informed consent be obtained for the use of all other agents. Before pregnancy the ratio of prandial to basal insulin is approximately 50%, but as efforts to achieve post-prandial glucose control intensify, prandial insulin can account for up to 70% of the total daily dose.

2.2.2 Basal insulin

Data concerning the safety and efficacy of basal analogues in pregnancy are lacking, prompting NICE to advocate Neutral Protamine Hagedorn (NPH) as the "first choice for long acting insulin during pregnancy". The 2008 NICE guidelines advise that women be offered CSII or insulin pump therapy if adequate glycaemic control is not obtained. However clinical and experimental data outside pregnancy suggest that basal insulin analogues may provide improved glycaemic control, with fewer severe and nocturnal hypoglycaemic episodes. In our clinic the majority of women enter pregnancy using basal analogues and are concerned that reverting to NPH will compromise glycaemic control and increase their risk of severe hypoglycaemia.

Results show no evidence of increased congenital malformation associated with basal analogue use (n = 335 pregnancies to date). We discuss the potential risks and benefits with women, documenting informed consent if they choose to continue. Risks include the lack of clinical experience and long-term use in pregnancy while potential benefits include reduced hypoglycaemia. An American study reported that glargine use was associated with significantly fewer macrosomic infants with lower rates of neonatal hyperbilirubinemia and hypoglycaemia. An Italian study (n = 30) suggested improved maternal glycaemic control during the first trimester with better fasting and 2 hours post-breakfast glucose levels during the first and second trimesters. The investigators questioned a potential association between glargine and shorter femoral length but it should be noted that the numbers of women in these and indeed all studies to date are small.

In our own study (n = 40) using serial 7-day CGM profiles, women using glargine during pregnancy spent 46% less time hypoglycaemic overnight compared to women using NPH (Figure 2.2). The time spent with BGL <3.5 mmol/l overnight for NPH compared to glargine was 13.1% (63 mins) versus 7.6% (36.3 mins) during the first trimester, 13.9% (67 mins) versus 8.1% (39 mins) during the second trimester and 15.2% (73 mins) versus 8.8% (42 mins) during the third trimester (p < 0.05).

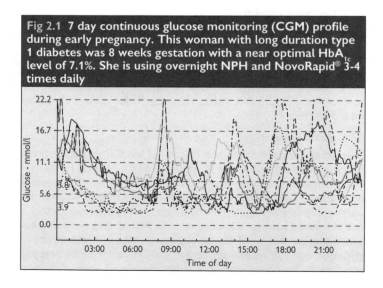

Fig 2.1 **7 day continuous glucose monitoring (CGM) profile during early pregnancy. This woman with long duration type 1 diabetes was 8 weeks gestation with a near optimal HbA$_{1c}$ level of 7.1%. She is using overnight NPH and NovoRapid® 3-4 times daily**

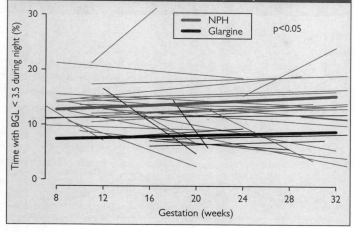

Fig 2.2 Overnight hypoglycaemia in women using NPH compared to glargine before bed. Thin lines represent the duration of time with overnight CGM glucose below 3.5 mmol/l in individual women while the thick lines represent the mean for NPH (grey) and glargine (black)

2.2.3 Continuous subcutaneous insulin infusion (CSII)

Pump therapy (CSII) more closely mimics physiological insulin secretion, with clinical experience and research evidence suggesting reduced episodes of severe hypoglycaemia and improved treatment satisfaction. However, widespread benefits on glycaemic control during pregnancy have not been realized, with recent reviews unable to demonstrate any difference between CSII and MDI therapy. The Cochrane review suggested a potential increase in infant birth weight associated with CSII, with a recent Polish study suggesting increased maternal weight gain in pump users. Pumps remain limited by user input, in particular frequency of blood glucose testing and accuracy of dose adjustment calculations, especially after meals and following physical activity. Therefore women using pumps require intensive multidisciplinary team support and frequent between clinic contacts to optimize insulin dose adjustment. Perhaps the increased use of continuous glucose monitoring in conjunction with pump use will help facilitate more precise dose adjustments but delays in insulin absorption (50 mins) and action (30 mins) contribute to the persistent difficulty achieving post-prandial targets. We are currently investigating the potential of closed loop therapy linking real-time continuous glucose monitoring, an individual insulin dose adjustment algorithm and insulin pump therapy to improve the day to day management of diabetes during pregnancy (Figure 2.3). Compared to conventional pump therapy, closed loop systems reduce glycaemic variability,

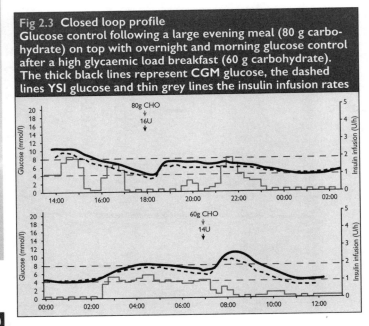

Fig 2.3 Closed loop profile
Glucose control following a large evening meal (80 g carbo-hydrate) on top with overnight and morning glucose control after a high glycaemic load breakfast (60 g carbohydrate). The thick black lines represent CGM glucose, the dashed lines YSI glucose and thin grey lines the insulin infusion rates

minimize hyper- and hypoglycaemic excursions and achieve near normoglycaemia overnight. Physiological studies to develop dose adjustment algorithms suitable for use in pregnancy are currently underway.

2.3 **Complications during pregnancy** (Table 2.2)

2.3.1 **Pre-eclampsia and pregnancy induced hypertension**
Although pre-pregnancy care improves early glycaemic control and reduces the risk of congenital malformation, it does not influence glycaemic control during later pregnancy and does not reduce the risks of macrocosmia and pre-eclampsia. These complications are related not to average glucose levels (mean blood glucose or HbA_{1c}) but to the hyperglycaemic spikes most commonly seen after meals and following treatment of hypoglycaemia as demonstrated in the 7-day CGM profile (Figure 2.1). Glycaemic control, nulliparity, diabetes duration and presence of microvascular disease (retinopathy and/or microalbuminuria) are well recognized risk factors for pre-eclampsia, the leading cause of preterm delivery.

In our experience it is poor glycaemic control during the second trimester, when placentation is underway, that is particularly

Table 2.2 Monitoring for complications of diabetes during pregnancy

Assessment	Booking	Trimester 2	Trimester 3	Post-partum
Glycaemic	HbA$_{1c}$ frequency/severity hypoglycaemia & hyperglycaemia	HbA$_{1c}$ frequency/severity Hypoglycaemia & hyperglycaemia	Frequency/severity Hypoglycaemia & hyperglycaemia	Hypoglycaemia frequency/severity
Retinal	Unless performed in past 6/12	16–20 weeks if previous retinopathy	28 weeks if no previous retinopathy	<6 months If retinopathy before/ during pregnancy
Renal	ACR, creatinine, lipids	16–20 weeks ACR, creatinine	28 weeks ACR, creatinine	<6 months
Congenital anomaly		18–20 weeks detailed ultrasound		
Fetal growth			4-weekly from 28–36 weeks	

implicated in the pathogenesis of pre-eclampsia in women with type 1 diabetes. Unlike pre-eclampisa it should be noted that the risk of pregnancy induced hypertension is not related to glycaemic control in women with type 1 diabetes, and seems to be more prevalent in women with type 2 diabetes, perhaps related to their increased age, parity, obesity and hyperlipidemia. Angiotensin-converting enzyme inhibitors and angiotensin-II receptor antagonists should be avoided and replaced by methyldopa and/or labetalol, which can be used under specialist supervision. While a target blood pressure of 135/85 mmHg is acceptable, more intensive glycaemic and blood pressure management improves pregnancy outcomes, and reduces risk of preterm delivery in women with hypertension and microalbuminuria.

2.3.2 Macrosomia

Macrosomia, defined as infant birth weight on or above the 90th centile for sex and gestational age, remains the commonest complication of pregnancy in women with diabetes. The risk of delivering a large for gestational age or macrosomic infant is approximately 50% both in women with type 1 and type 2 diabetes. This leads to increased risk of maternal birth trauma, perineal lacerations, labour complications and delivery by caesarean section. For their infants, there are immediate complications of intracranial haemorrhage, shoulder dystocia, neonatal hypoglycaemia, jaundice, and respiratory distress as well as the longer-term health risks of insulin resistance, obesity, and type 2 diabetes. Although educational approaches incorporating additional glucose testing after meals to improve glycaemic control during the second and third trimesters have shown potential, there has been very little progress in reducing the birth weight of infants born to mothers with diabetes in recent decades.

Novel methods of continuous glucose monitoring (CGM) provide detailed data on the magnitude and duration of glucose excursions particularly overnight and after meals.

We evaluated the role of supplementary continuous glucose monitoring in women with pregestational diabetes attending routine antenatal clinics. Although small (n = 71) this randomized clinical study documented improvements both in maternal glycaemic control and in neonatal health outcomes, with lower infant birth weight and significantly reduced risk of macrosomia in infants of mothers using supplementary continuous glucose monitoring. Real time CGM offers the possibility of acting immediately to correct and/or prevent glucose excursions. Pilot interventions suggest 20–30% reductions in glucose excursions during short-term use with a large randomized study demonstrating significant reductions in HbA_{1c} (approximately 0.5%) associated with sustained sensor use (>6 days/week). One small study (n = 12) suggested benefits using real time continuous glucose monitoring with mean birth weight of infants in mothers using continuous glucose monitoring of 3,309 g compared to 3,688 g for infants in the control group. The results from a large scale study in the Netherlands will provide further evidence regarding the effectiveness of continuous glucose monitoring during pregnancy.

2.3.3 Monitoring for complications of diabetes

2.3.3.1 Glycaemic assessment

This includes documentation of the average number of daily blood glucose tests, typically 7–10 per day, if performed before and 1-hour after meals, before bed and following the diagnosis and treatment of hypoglycaemic episodes. If there is suspected nocturnal hypoglycaemia or elevated fasting blood glucose levels we recommend additional overnight testing between 02.00–04.00 hr. To adjust overnight basal rates for insulin pump users at least two to three overnight tests per week are required. We advise that blood glucose meters be downloaded at each visit to document the mean blood glucose level and the frequency and severity of hypo- and hyperglycaemic excursions. In addition the presence or absence of severe hypoglycaemia (defined as needing third party assistance) should be documented at each visit. Insulin pump users commonly use an electronic diary to allow for more detailed documentation of insulin dose adjustments.

For assessment of average glycaemic control, we perform routine HbA$_{1c}$ testing at booking, between 16–20 weeks' and at 28 weeks' gestation, although the latter is not supported by the recent NICE guidelines. However women are having bloods taken for renal and full blood count review and while a satisfactory HbA$_{1c}$ level may not inform clinical decisions, HbA$_{1c}$ levels >7% during the third trimester are associated with increased perinatal morbidity and mortality and warrant increased obstetric surveillance. Newer markers of intermediate glycaemic control are currently being evaluated and may be of value in the future, particularly if they accurately reflect post-prandial glucose excursions.

2.3.3.2 Retinal assessment

In women who have attended pre-pregnancy care, retinal assessment digital retinal photography (with mydriasis using tropicamide) should have been performed during the 6 months prior to pregnancy. If this is entirely normal the repeat measurement can be delayed to 28 weeks' gestation. However in women without recent retinal review this should be performed as soon as possible after pregnancy is confirmed, and repeated at 16–20 weeks if there is any evidence of retinopathy and at 28 weeks if normal. Ophthalmology input is recommended for women with any degree of retinopathy before and during pregnancy, with repeat assessment within 6 months post-partum to document whether changes during pregnancy have resolved. The NICE guidelines provide absolute clarity that diabetic retinopathy is not a contraindication to rapid optimization of glycaemic control during pregnancy and does not preclude a vaginal delivery.

2.3.3.3 Renal assessment

We perform a renal assessment at booking to document baseline blood pressure, urinary albumin excretion, albumin creatinine ratio (ACR), serum creatinine and lipid profile. In women with microalbuminuria (urinary albumin 30–300 mg), ACR >3.5 mg/mmol, or creatinine >120 µmol/l at booking, meticulous attention to glycaemic and blood pressure control is required. In normotensive women, urinary albumin and serum creatinine measurements are repeated at 16–20 and at 28 weeks' gestation. In the presence of microalbuminuria and/or hypertension we titrate treatment to maintain BP < 135/85 and urinary albumin <300 mg/24hr. The preferred anti-hypertensive agents used during pregnancy are methyldopa and labetalol with angiotensin-converting enzyme (ACE) inhibitors used only with written consent in exceptional cases, when the potential benefits may outweigh the risks. Thromboprophylaxis and nephrologist input are considered in all women with incipient nephropathy.

2.3.3.4 Screening for congenital anomaly

Women should be offered a detailed ultrasound examination at 18–20 weeks focusing in particular on the neural tube structures, the fetal heart and outflow tracts.

2.3.3.5 Fetal growth assessment

Ultrasound monitoring of fetal growth and amniotic fluid volume, with careful documentation of the fetal growth centile and abdominal circumference is performed every 4 weeks from 28 to 36 weeks. In women with pregestational diabetes (unlike their counterparts with gestational diabetes), a normal growth trajectory at 28 weeks makes significant later growth acceleration and an extremely large for gestational age infant less likely. However there is no evidence that growth acceleration at 28 weeks can be significantly reduced by tightening glycaemic control later in the third trimester. We therefore focus on supporting women to achieve the tightest possible post-prandial glycaemic control throughout the second trimester and before the development of acceleration at 28 weeks.

Further reading

Farrar D, Tuffnell DJ, West J (2007). Continuous subcutaneous insulin infusion versus multiple daily injections of insulin for pregnant women with diabetes. *Cochrane Database Syst Rev* **3**: CD005542.

Hovorka R (2006). Continuous glucose monitoring and closed-loop systems. *Diabet Med* **23**: 1–12.

Macintosh MC, Fleming KM, Bailey JM, *et al.* (2006). Perinatal mortality and congenital anomalies in babies of women with type 1 or type 2 diabetes in England, Wales, and Northern Ireland: population based study. *BMJ* **333**: 177.

Murphy HR, Rayman G, Duffield K, *et al.* (2007). Changes in the glycemic profiles of women with type 1 and type 2 diabetes during pregnancy. *Diabetes Care* **30**: 2785–91.

Murphy HR, Rayman G, Lewis K, *et al.* (2008). Effectiveness of continuous glucose monitoring in pregnant women with diabetes: randomised clinical trial. *BMJ* **337**: a1680.

National Institute for Health and Clinical Excellence (NICE) (2008). Diabetes in pregnancy. *Management of diabetes and its complications from pre-conception to the postnatal period. NICE clinical guideline* **63**. NICE, London.

Temple RC, Aldridge VJ, Murphy HR (2006). Prepregnancy care and pregnancy outcomes in women with type 1 diabetes. *Diabetes Care* **29**: 1744–9.

Chapter 3

Gestational diabetes risk factors, detection and diagnosis

Robert Lindsay

> **Key points**
> - Gestational diabetes has a number of risk factors in common with type 2 diabetes including family history of type 2 diabetes, obesity and overweight, ethnicity, age, and previous macrosomia.
> - There has long been controversy over the diagnosis of gestational diabetes which new international criteria may help to resolve.
> - In any screening programme consideration should be given to the need to detect previously undiagnosed type 2 diabetes in early pregnancy.

3.1 Introduction

While it has long been apparent that there is a relationship between higher maternal blood sugar and complications in pregnancy—notably macrosomia, shoulder dystocia, preeclampsia, and neonatal hypoglycaemia—there has been controversy over the best method for screening and diagnosis of gestational diabetes. Gestational diabetes is usually defined as diabetes with first onset or recognition in pregnancy (WHO, 1999). Under this definition women with pre-existing but previously undiagnosed diabetes (usually type 2 diabetes) or who develop type 1 diabetes during pregnancy are included as gestational diabetes. That said, by far the greatest number of cases relate to a rise in blood glucose during pregnancy in response to the well-documented worsening of insulin resistance during gestation. Glucose tolerance then usually returns to normal after delivery. It is known that the risk of such a deterioration in glucose tolerance is related to underlying risk of type 2 diabetes with family history of type 2 diabetes, obesity, ethnicity, age, and previous macrosomia acting as risk factors for the condition. Difficulty has arisen in defining the best method for screening for gestational diabetes and, as the risk of adverse effects such as macrosomia describe a continuum, the most effective level at which gestational diabetes might be diagnosed. While there have been many different criteria and screening systems we will describe those defined by the most recent NICE guidelines (NICE, 2008) in 2008, International Association of Diabetes And Pregnancy Study Groups (IADPSG) in 2010 (IADPSG, 2010), and Scottish Intercollegiate Guidelines Network (SIGN) in 2010 (SIGN, 2010) after a brief historical note outlining some of the previous methods and approaches in less detail.

3.2 Gestational diabetes: a historical note

While the adverse consequences of gestational diabetes to the off-spring have been noted for some time, some of the original definitions of gestational diabetes, following the pioneering work of Carpenter and Coustan, related risk of glucose intolerance during pregnancy not to fetal or newborn outcomes but rather to later risk of type 2 diabetes in the mother. This was unsatisfactory and perhaps contributed to the lingering concern of some obstetricians that diabetologists' interest was the early detection of metabolic disease in the mother rather than outcomes for the child.

Historically the literature on gestational diabetes was often difficult to interpret as a variety of approaches were taken and diagnostic levels were not always tied to fetal outcomes. In the United States, screening was achieved using a 50 g oral glucose load with a single blood test taken at 1 hour (the oral glucose challenge test—OGCT). Subsequently in women with a 1 hour blood glucose above threshold (usually 7.8 mmol/l) proceeded to a diagnostic test with an oral glucose tolerance test (OGTT) using a 100 g glucose load. By contrast in the United Kingdom and much of Europe screening, if carried out, was by risk factors, random glucose, urinalysis for glycosuria or fasting glucose, and the definitive test was the 75 g OGTT. Happily while differences have not been entirely resolved there has been a consensus developing. There appears to be increasing agreement with regard to use of 75 g of glucose as the diagnostic test. Thus from 1998 the American Diabetes Association have included provision for a single 75g OGTT as an alternative to the more traditional 50 g OGCT and subsequent 100 g OGTT (ADA, 2004). The most recent IADPSG consensus is based around the 75 g OGTT for diagnosis. Instructions for carrying out the 75 g OGTT are included in Table 3.1.

The level of glucose used to determine gestational diabetes has also differed around the world. As detailed the original definitions

Table 3.1 The 75 g oral glucose tolerance test (1)

- The OGTT should be administered in the morning after at least three days of unrestricted diet (greater than 150 g of carbohydrate daily) and usual physical activity
- The test should be preceded by an overnight fast of 8–14 hours, during which water may be drunk
- Smoking is not permitted during the test
- The subject should drink 75 g of anhydrous glucose or 82.5 g of glucose monohydrate in 250–300 ml of water over the course of 5 minutes[†]
- Timing of the test is from the beginning of the drink
- Blood samples must be collected 2 hours after the test load.

[†] In practice commercial glucose solutions, e.g. 410 ml standard Lucozade® are often substituted.

of gestational diabetes in the United States were based on the mother's later risk of type 2 diabetes rather than features in the fetus or newborn. In 1998 the World Health Organization published its influential report on the diagnosis and classification of diabetes mellitus (WHO, 1999). Notably they proposed that the definition comprised the categories of impaired glucose tolerance (fasting venous plasma glucose <7.0 mmol/l and 2 hour glucose 7.8–11.0 mmol/l) and diabetes (fasting venous plasma glucose ≥7.0 mmol/l or 2 hour glucose ≥11.1 mmol/l) in the non-pregnant state. Outwith pregnancy the levels of blood glucose used to diagnose diabetes are based predominantly on those levels above which a greatly increased risk of microvascular complications (retinopathy, nephropathy and neuropathy) are observed (WHO, 1999). There is therefore a logic to the level chosen as the diagnosis of diabetes carries with it the need for entry of patients into screening programmes for microvascular disease. As will be discussed later the continuous nature of the relationship between maternal glucose and risk of complications does not allow the level at which gestational diabetes should be diagnosed to be determined in such a straightforward way. The rationale for inclusion of the categories of impaired glucose tolerance and diabetes as gestational diabetes in the 1999 WHO report is less apparent. For example, there is a discordance between the fasting level (≥7.0 mmol/l) which represents a very extreme fasting glucose in the pregnant population and the diagnostic level 2 hours after the oral glucose tolerance test (≥11.1 mmol/l), which lies around the 90th percentile for 2 hour blood glucose between 24 and 28 weeks of pregnancy. By contrast criteria bases on the 100 g OGTT were different again (usually two or more of fasting glucose ≥5.3 mmol/l, 1 hour ≥ 10.0 mmol/l, 2 hour ≥8.6 mmol/l or 3 hour ≥7.8 mmol/l). Taken together there was a great deal of confusion and unsatisfactory literature due to difficulty in comparing studies from different

29

health care systems and much need for the attempts at consensus found after the Hyperglycaemia and Pregnancy Outcomes (HAPO) study.

3.3 Physiology of glucose tolerance in pregnancy

Normal pregnancy is associated with a number of changes in glucose tolerance and intermediate metabolism more generally. Most notably pregnancy is an insulin resistant state. Data from the gold standard of assessment of insulin action—the euglycaemic glucose clamp—demonstrate that insulin action reduces as pregnancy progresses. Clinically this is reflected in increases in insulin requirement in women with type 1 diabetes of on average 60% in insulin doses as pregnancy progresses to maintain euglycaemia. The change in insulin requirement reflects the alteration in the hormonal milieu experienced as pregnancy progresses. There appear to be important roles of placental products in particular, with human placental lactogen and placental production of tumour necrosis alpha (TNF-alpha) appearing key in the development of insulin resistance (Kirwan et al., 2002). At the same time there are changes in fasting glucose likely reflecting an increased uptake of glucose by the feto-placental unit. Fasting glucose in normal women is relatively low in pregnancy. Fasting venous plasma glucose was on average 4.5 mmol/l (standard deviation 0.4 mmol/l) in the HAPO study while studies using home monitoring of capillary blood glucose suggest that average fasting capillary glucose readings in are as low as 56 mg/dl (3.0 mmol/l) in healthy, lean, normal glucose tolerant women in the third trimester of pregnancy (Paretti et al., 2001).

There are a number of other important metabolic changes. Blood lipids increase in pregnancy, teleologically to aid transfer of nutrients to the feto-placental unit with a subsequent increase in total cholesterol, HDL cholesterol, LDL cholesterol and triglycerides. There are increases in circulating amino acids and likely small increases in circulating lactate. In terms of acid-base balance pregnancy is usually described as being a state of mild respiratory alkalosis, it is believed that this results directly form effects of circulating maternal oestradiol on respiratory centres with resulting small falls in pCO_2 and bicarbonate. The latter fall may be of importance in interpretation of venous bicarbonate where women are assessed for potential diabetic ketoacidosis.

Finally as part of the change of plasma lipids there is an increased tendency to metabolise fats—a state known as accelerated starvation or accelerated ketogenesis (Metzger et al., 1982). This has been described for some time and in essence involves an earlier shift postprandially to mobilization of fat stores. The clinical result of this is that ketogenesis will occur after a shorter fast in pregnancy than out of pregnancy—leading to the observation that up to 30% of women will elaborate ketones on urine testing in the morning. For women with type 1 diabetes the effect is an earlier progression to ketogenesis and ketoacidosis if insulin doses are withheld or delayed.

3.4 **Adverse consequences of gestational diabetes**

The adverse consequences of gestational diabetes have been known for some time but most clearly delineated by the multinational multicentre Hyperglycaemia and Pregnancy Outcome Study (HAPO). This study examined over 23,000 women with glucose tolerance short of frank diabetes in pregnancy. Thus women were included if fasting glucose was less than 5.8 mmol/l and two hour glucose was less than 11.1 mmol. Notably around 1.7% of women were *not* included in the study because of a raised fasting or 2 hour value at baseline. A further 1.2% of women were omitted from the study due to raised random glucose (>8.9 mmol/l) later in pregnancy. These mothers were excluded as the results of blood glucose in the HAPO study were otherwise blinded and it was felt unethical to not transmit results at this level to clinicians to start treatment. Thus the HAPO population excludes both women with known pregestational diabetes but also potentially 2.9% of the normal population with the highest glucose levels during pregnancy.

The HAPO study has indicated a continuous relationship of fasting, 1 hour and 2 hour glucose after a 75 g OGTT with a variety of pregnancy outcomes. For the primary outcomes of the HAPO study there was a continuous graded relationship with likelihood of macrosomia, cord insulin >90th percentile, clinical neonatal hypoglycaemia and caesarean section (Figure 3.1) (Metzger et al., 2008). Later publications from the HAPO study indicated a continuous relationship of maternal glucose with neonatal adiposity (HAPO, 2009). Of all of the HAPO outcomes neonatal hypoglycaemia arguably did show a threshold effect that is a "step up" in risk in those at the highest levels of maternal blood glucose.

The HAPO investigators also examined a range of other important outcomes. Of these secondary outcomes shoulder dystocia and pre-eclampsia were positively associated with maternal fasting and post-challenge blood glucose while pre-term delivery, hyperbilirubinaemia and intensive neonatal care were related to post-challenge but not fasting glucose. The study was not powered for, and did not show, any significant relationship with perinatal mortality—perhaps

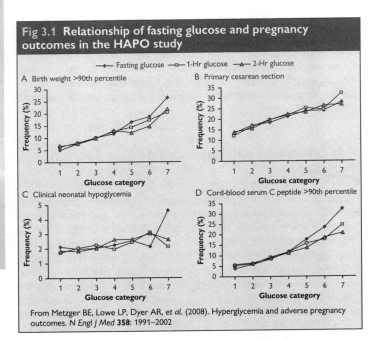

Fig 3.1 Relationship of fasting glucose and pregnancy outcomes in the HAPO study

From Metzger BE, Lowe LP, Dyer AR, et al. (2008). Hyperglycemia and adverse pregnancy outcomes. N Engl J Med **358**: 1991–2002

reflecting the exclusion of mothers at the highest level of blood glucose.

The HAPO data are largely in keeping with previous results in the literature. Most notably there has not been a convincing relationship of gestational diabetes to stillbirth or perinatal mortality in the past with only a few studies suggesting such a relationship.

3.5 Screening and diagnosis of gestational diabetes

The HAPO study has provided an important new platform for defining the risk that can be attributed to maternal glucose—as assessed by the 75 g OGTT. Most importantly, since the relationship of maternal glucose to outcomes is a continuum the exact level at which gestational diabetes is diagnosed can only be agreed by consensus. The approaches of the American Diabetes Association (ADA), International Association of Diabetes and Pregnancy Study Groups (IADPSG), NICE and Scottish Intercollegiate Guidelines Network (SIGN) are at present different but it is hoped that there will be convergence at least in use of the 75 g OGTT and the diagnostic criteria proposed by the IADPSG. Screening systems may always be divergent—not least as the underlying risk of diabetes in different populations will differ depending on ethnicity and the prevalence of risk factors.

One notable feature of the newer screening strategies is the acknowledgement of the importance of detecting pre-existing (pre-gestational but undiagnosed) diabetes early in pregnancy. The IADPSG consensus suggests measurement of fasting plasma glucose haemoglobin A1C, or random plasma glucose at the first antenatal visit. Overt diabetes is diagnosed if fasting venous plasma glucose is ≥7.0 mmol/l or HbA$_{1c}$ is ≥6.5% or random venous plasma glucose ≥11.1 mmol/l. This newer emphasis on early detection of pre-existing diabetes reflects the secular increase in type 2 diabetes in turn driven by adverse diet and lifestyle. This has greatly increased the likely number of women detected with pre-existing diabetes in early pregnancy. Such women should be offered appropriate screening for risk of congenital anomaly and diabetes complications in the mother, and early biochemical screening allows this. The IADPSG consensus suggests that early pregnancy screening occurs either in all or only high risk women depending on the population and underlying diabetes risk out of pregnancy.

For screening in later pregnancy most previous systems propose some stratification by non-biochemical risk factors (Table 3.2). Specific risk factors proposed by ADA and NICE are presented in Table 3.3. There is a weakness in this approach. First it should be noted that the panel of risk factors proposed by NICE include approximately 40–50% of the population in countries such as the UK—so a large group of women are still required to go through biochemical screening. Secondly it is acknowledged in the NICE report that such risk factors are relatively insensitive—that is cases that would have been picked up on universal screening will be missed with this selective approach. By contrast the IADPSG suggest universal screening—so that all women have a 75 g OGTT if they have not already been diagnosed with diabetes in pregnancy by 24–28 weeks. While this approach will be more familiar to countries who already a screening biochemical test—the 50 g oral glucose challenge test—in all or most women universal screening will be a major change in practice for countries, like the UK, where only a minority of women have traditionally had some form of glucose challenge in pregnancy.

Diagnostic criteria are summarized in Table 3.2. As detailed in the discussion on HAPO the continuous relationship of maternal glucose to outcomes means that there is no immediately obvious "cut off" at which gestational diabetes should be diagnosed. This however does not mean that the choice is arbitrary. It is clearly possible to establish a level of maternal glucose defining increased risk of macrosomia,

Table 3.2 Screening and diagnostic schema

	ADA (2004)	NICE (2008)	IADPSG (2010)	SIGN (2010)
Initial screening	By risk factors (Table 3.3)	By risk factors (Table 3.3)	All women screened at 24–28 weeks	By risk factors (Table 3.3), low risk women offered fasting glucose at 24–28 weeks
Biochemical screening test	50 g oral glucose challenge test with 100 g OGTT if 1 hour value >7.8 mmol/l (two step approach)	-	-	-
Diagnostic test	100 g OGTT (two step) OR 75 g OGTT (one step)	75 g OGTT	75 g OGTT	75 g OGTT
Timing of diagnostic test	24–28 weeks	24–28 weeks	24–28 weeks	24–28 weeks
Diagnostic criteria	Two or more of Fasting ≥5.3 mmol/l OR 1 hour ≥10.0 mmol/l OR 2 hour ≥8.6 mmol/l OR 3 hour ≥7.8 mmol/l	Fasting ≥7.0 mmol/l OR 2 hour ≥11.1 mmol/l	Fasting ≥5.1 mmol/l OR 1 hour ≥10.0 mmol/l OR 2 hour ≥8.5 mmol/l	Fasting ≥5.1 mmol/l OR 1 hour ≥10.0 mmol/l OR 2 hour ≥8.5 mmol/l

ADA = American Diabetes Association
NICE = National Institute for Health and Clinical Excellence
IADPSG = International Association of Diabetes and Pregnancy Study Groups
SIGN = Scottish Intercollegiate Guidelines Network

Table 3.3 Risk factors used to select women for screening for gestational diabetes

	ADA 2000	NICE 2008
Application	Any one of the risk factors present then biochemical screening should occur	Any one of the risk factors present then biochemical screening should occur
	Age ≥25 years Weight not "normal" before pregnancy Not member of ethnic group with low risk of GDM History of diabetes in first degree relative History of abnormal glucose tolerance History of poor obstetric outcome	BMI more than 30 kg/m² Previous macrosomic baby weighing 4.5 kg or more Previous gestational diabetes Family history of diabetes (first degree relative with diabetes) Family origin with a high prevalence of diabetes: • South Asian (specifically women whose country of family origin is India, Pakistan or Bangladesh) • black Caribbean • Middle Eastern (specifically women whose country of family origin is Saudi Arabia, United Arab Emirates, Iraq, Jordan, Syria, Oman, Qatar, Kuwait, Lebanon or Egypt).

caesarean section, pre-eclampsia and other adverse outcomes. The key demonstration that treatment of gestational diabetes improved outcomes (summarized in Chapter 4) has meant that we can more clearly now define the population at risk and likely benefit of intervention. Ultimately some of the decision making around the diagnosis of gestational diabetes may now involve health economic analysis as to the costs of case detection and overall benefits of treatment. Nevertheless it is hoped that there will be a widespread adoption of the IADPSG criteria for the diagnosis of gestational diabetes. These were achieved by consensus and based on the level of blood glucose above which key adverse outcomes (birthweight, cord C-peptide, and percent body fat >90th percentile) achieved an odds ratio of 1.75 fold compared to mothers with average glucose. This results in an increase in these key outcomes in the group testing positive for gestational diabetes (Table 3.4). Use of these criteria in combination with universal oral glucose tolerance testing would be expected to result in around 16–20% of women being diagnosed with gestational diabetes—a major change for most health care systems. Application of the criteria defines a population at increased risk of macrosomia,

Table 3.4 **Adverse outcomes in women above and below diagnostic criteria in the HAPO population**

Outcome	FPG,1-hr and 2-hr OGTT values all <threshold	FPG and/or 1-hr and/or 2-hr OGTT values >threshold
Birthweight > 90th percentile	8.3%	16.2%**
Cord C-peptide > 90th percentile	6.7%	17.5%**
Percent body fat > 90th percentile	8.5%	16.6%**
Pre-eclampsia	4.5%	9.1%**
Preterm delivery (<37 weeks)	6.4%	9.4%**
Primary caesarean section	16.8%	24.4**
Shoulder dystocia and/or birth injury	1.3%	1.8%**
Clinical neonatal hypoglycemia	1.9%	2.7%**
Hyperbilirubinemia	8.0%	10.0%**
Intensive neonatal care	7.8%	9.1%**

* Thresold values: FPG ≥ 5.1 mmol/l (92 mg/dl), 1-hr PG ≥ 10.0 mmol/l (180 mg/dl), 2-hr ≥ 8.5 mmol/l (153 mg/dl)
* Difference between groups siginificant at p < 0.01
** Difference between groups siginificant at p < 0.001
(From Metzger BE, Lowe LP, Dyer AR, et al. (2000). Hyperglycemia and adverse pregnancy outcomes. *N Engl J Med* **358**: 1991–2002)

hyperinsulinaemia and increased neonatal adiposity although predictably these conditions may also occur in women not fulfilling the criteria (Table 3.4). Importantly analysis of the HAPO dataset also shows that pre-eclampsia preterm delivery, shoulder dystocia are also increased by 30–100% (Table 3.4).

Further reading

American Diabetes Association (2004). Clinical practice recomendation: gestational diabetes. *Diabetes Care* **27**, S1.

HAPO Study Cooperative Research Group (2009). Hyperglycemia and Adverse Pregnancy Outcome (HAPO) Study: associations with neonatal anthropometrics. *Diabetes* **58**: 453–9.

International Association of Diabetes and Pregnancy Study Groups Consensus Panel (2010). International Association of Diabetes and Pregnancy Study

Groups recommendations on the diagnosis and classification of hyperglycemia in pregnancy. *Diabetes Care* **33**: 676–82.

Kirwan JP, Hauguel-De Mouzon S, Lepercq J, *et al.* (2002). TNF-alpha is a predictor of insulin resistance in human pregnancy. *Diabetes* **51**: 2207–13.

Metzger BE, Ravnikar V, Vileisis RA, Freinkel N (1982). "Accelerated starvation" and the skipped breakfast in late normal pregnancy. *Lancet* **1**: 588–92.

Metzger BE, Lowe LP, Dyer AR, *et al.* (2008). Hyperglycemia and adverse pregnancy outcomes. *N Engl J Med* **358**: 1991–2002.

National Institute for Health and Clinical Excellence (2008). Diabetes in pregnancy: management of diabetes and its complications from pre-conception to the postnatal period. *NICE clinical guideline* **63**. NICE, London.

Parretti E, Mecacci F, Papini M, *et al.* (2001). Third-trimester maternal glucose levels from diurnal profiles in nondiabetic pregnancies: correlation with sonographic parameters of fetal growth. *Diabetes Care* **24**: 1319–23.

Scottish Intercollegiate Guidelines Network (2010). *Management of diabetes: a national clinical guideline*, **116**. SIGN, Edinburgh.

World Health Organization (1999). *Definition, diagnosis and classification of diabetes mellitus and its complications*. WHO, Geneva.

Chapter 4

Gestational diabetes: management in pregnancy

Robert Lindsay

Key points

- Two recent large trials demonstrate that detection and management of gestational diabetes improves outcomes.
- While gestational diabetes is predominantly managed by diet and lifestyle change use of glibenclamide and metformin can be considered as second-line therapy.

4.1 Background

As discussed in Chapter 3 there has been substantial historical controversy over the diagnostic criteria for gestational diabetes and even whether screening itself was appropriate. An added element of clinical doubt was raised due to the lack of randomized control trials examining the effect of treatment on outcomes—many previous studies being observational in design. Concern was also raised that labelling women as having gestational diabetes might result in adverse outcomes—such as increased rates of caesarean section—as clinicians responded to a perceived increased in risk with a more conservative obstetric approach. In keeping with the state of the evidence at the time, NICE concluded in 2002 that there was insufficient evidence to advocate universal screening for gestational diabetes (Scott et al., 2002) although they also observed that there were clearly some women in whom maternal hyperglycaemia was causing adverse fetal outcomes. Since that time two major trials published in 2005 (Crowther et al., 2005) and 2009 (Landon et al., 2009) have examined the effect on pregnancy outcomes of detection and management of gestational diabetes. Randomized control trials in gestational diabetes have also examined the efficacy of metformin (Rowan et al., 2008) adding to the older literature on the use of glibenclamide (glyburide) (Langer et al., 2000). Collectively this new evidence clearly demonstrates that fetal growth can be modified by glucose-lowering therapies and that treatment strategies starting with oral hypoglycaemic agents (metformin or glibenclamide) but often involving progression to insulin are as successful but not superior as insulin alone.

4.2 Management of gestational diabetes: the rationale for treatment

Two large randomized controlled trials have investigated the effects of screening, diagnosis, and treatment of gestational diabetes. The design of both trials were broadly similar. Women had biochemical screening and were either randomized to blood glucose lowering therapy—starting with diet, lifestyle and glucose monitoring and progressing to insulin therapy as needed—or the results of their glucose tolerance tests were kept blinded. In both cases women with the highest levels of blood glucose either at baseline or if detected in routine follow up were excluded.

The Australian Carbohydrate Intolerance Study in Pregnant Women (ACHOIS) reported in 2005 (Crowther et al., 2005). Women diagnosed with gestational diabetes at 24–34 weeks of gestation were randomized to either dietary advice, blood glucose monitoring and where indicated insulin therapy (the intervention group), or routine care. Treatment of gestational diabetes reduced birth weight by 147 g and reduced rates of macrosomia (birth weight >4 kg) from 21% to 10% and large for gestational age (LGA >90th percentile) from 22% to 13%. The primary composite outcome (serious perinatal outcomes: death, shoulder dystocia, bone fracture and nerve palsy) was also significantly reduced from 4% to 1% (Crowther et al., 2005).

More recently the Maternal Fetal Medicines Unit Network (MFMU) trial of treatment of mild gestational diabetes used a similar design and intervention to ACHOIS but entry levels of glycaemia were lower (fasting glucose <5.3 mmol/l and two or three post load glucoses above established thresholds) (Landon et al., 2009). The primary outcome was not achieved (a composite of perinatal mortality, hypoglycaemia, hyperbilirubinaemia, neonatal hyperinsulinaemia, and birth trauma) but there were significant reductions in birth weight (by 106 g), birth weight >4 kg (5.9% vs. 14.3%), large for gestational age (7.1% vs. 14.5%) and caesarean section (26.9% intervention vs. 33.8% in control) with treatment of gestational diabetes.

Table 4.1 Relative risk for adverse outcomes in ACHOIS and MFMU

	ACHOIS	MFMU
Primary outcome	↓ 0.33 (0.14–0.75) (P = 0.01)	↔ 0.87 (0.72–1.07) NS
Large for gestational age	↓ 0.62 (0.47–0.81) (P <0.001)	↓ 0.49 (32–0.76) (P <0.001)
Macrosomia birth weight >4 kg	↓ 0.47 (0.34–0.64) (P <0.001)	↓ 0.41 (0.26–0.66) (P <0.001)
Neonatal fat mass	–	↓ (P = 0.003)
NICU admission	↑ 1.13 (1.03–1.23) (P = 0.04)	↔ 0.77 (0.51–1.18) (P = NS)
Shoulder dystocia	↔ 0.46 (0.19–1.10) (P = NS)	↓ 0.37 (0.14–0.97) (P = 0.02)
Induction	↑ 1.36 (1.15–1.62) (P <0.001)	↔ 1.02 (0.81–1.29) (P = NS)
Pre-eclampsia	↓ 0.70 (0.51–0.95) (P = 0.02)	↓ 0.46 (0.22–0.97) (P = 0.02)
Caesarean section	↔ 0.97 (0.81–1.16) (P = NS)	↓ 0.79 (0.64–0.99) (P = 0.02)

All figures are given as the relative risk (95% confidence intervals) in the intervention vs. control arms of the respective studies. NS = not significant

In comparing the two studies it would appear that women in the MFMU study likely had somewhat lower levels of blood glucose. Rates of large for gestational age babies were higher in the control (untreated) group of the ACHOIS study than MFMU (22% and 14.5% respectively). It is clear that detection and treatment of gestational diabetes reduced birth weight along with rates of large for gestational age and macrosomia (Table 4.1). Taken together it is apparent that shoulder dystocia and pre-eclampsia are reduced while there were increases in rates of induction and neonatal nursery admissions in the ACHOIS trial only. This may have related to clinical practice rather than underlying morbidity but is an important outcome both for the mother and potentially for healthcare costs. Conversely the MFMU trial showed a reduction in caesarean section rates (Table 4.1).

4.3 Dietary and lifestyle intervention

The key first step in the management of gestational diabetes is dietary intervention. There are relatively few randomized control trials.

The MFMU study recommended dietary therapy in keeping with ADA guidelines with a carbohydrate-controlled meal plan promoting "appropriate gestational weight gain, achievement and maintenance of normoglycemia, and absence of ketosis." In ACHOIS patients had individualized dietary advice along the same lines. There is a literature examining the beneficial effects of exercise on gestational diabetes. This should be encouraged as there are benefits not only in terms of glycaemic control but also more generally on women's health in pregnancy. Nevertheless in clinical practice women often find it difficult to increase their exercise particularly in later pregnancy.

4.4 Glycaemic monitoring and blood glucose targets

Both the MFMU and ACHOIS studies monitored blood glucose four times daily fasting and two hours after meals. In ACHOIS this was completed for the first two weeks and then at rotating times as long as targets were being met. Strategies for institution and increase in insulin therapy followed prevailing guideline advice of the time and are summarized in Table 4.2. There is a paucity of randomized evidence supporting modifications of these approaches. A single RCT does support improved outcomes using post-prandial rather than pre-prandial testing (de Veciana et al., 1995), however it is difficult to assess whether these improvements also reflected subtly tighter targets in the post-prandial group. Pragmatically it would appear appropriate to follow the protocols of ACHOIS or MFMU.

There is also an open question over the extent to which glycaemic targets should be individualized. A number of trials would support the contention that tighter glycaemic control will exert a greater effect on fetal growth. For example in the study of Rowan et al. of metformin therapy in gestational diabetes (see Section 4.5), the

Table 4.2 Glycaemic targets in ACHOIS and MFMU		
	ACHOIS	**MFMU**
Fasting capillary blood glucose	3.5–5.5 mmol/l	<5.3 mmol/l
Two hour capillary blood glucose	<7.0 mmol/l (<8.0 mmol/l after 35 weeks)	<6.7 mmol/l
Criterion for institution or increase in insulin	Two values above target in a two week period or one value >9.0 mmol/l	If "majority of fasting values or post prandial values between study visits elevated"

achieved level of blood glucose (non-randomized) within the treated group was associated with improved outcomes (Rowan *et al.*, 2010). The lowest risk of complications—including birth weight >4 kg, prematurity, pre-eclampsia and neonatal hypoglycaemia—occurred with fasting capillary glucose levels ≤4.9 mmol/l and 2-h postprandial glucose 5.9–6.4 mmol/l—which are below conventional targets. There is also a suggestion that overtight glycaemic control might increase the risk of women delivering small for gestational age babies.

Such information supports the hypothesis that "fetal based strategies" might be favourable. Fetal growth and in particular abdominal circumference are used to try to select women for more or less tight glycaemic control. It is known that ultrasound assessment is predictive of complications at delivery (caesarean section, shoulder dystocia, birth trauma) and abdominal circumference correlates with the degree of fetal insulinaemia (Schaefer-Graf *et al.*, 2003). Four randomized control trials have used ultrasound (abdominal circumference ≥75th or ≥70th percentiles) to select women for insulin initiation or intensification. The trials have used differing levels of less intensive (where abdominal circumference <70th or 75th percentiles) and more intensive (where abdominal circumference >75th or 70th percentile) glycaemic management. These trials have been associated with either equivalent outcomes (Buchanan *et al.*, 1994, Kjos *et al.*, 2001, Schaefer-Graf *et al.*, 2004) or improved outcomes (birth weight, macrosomia, rates of large for gestational age) in women with gestational diabetes (Bonomo *et al.*, 2004). Improved outcomes were also found with ultrasound assessment at 28 weeks and early initiation of insulin (Rossi *et al.*, 2000). Taken together these trials suggest the fetal abdominal circumference can be used to select women for more or less intensive glycaemic control.

43

4.5 Management of gestational diabetes: oral hypoglycaemics

Where dietary intervention fails to control blood sugar it is appropriate to consider pharmacological therapy. In the past this has been predominantly insulin-based and this will be discussed in due course. More recently both the sulphonylureas glibenclamide and metformin have been investigated for use in gestational diabetes.

Traditionally sulphonylureas were not used in pregnancy. Sulphonylureas act to increase insulin secretion by direct effects on the pancreatic beta cell sulphonylurea receptor. Early sulphonylureas were found to cross the placenta. Since one of the aims of treatment of gestational diabetes is reduction of fetal hyperinsulinaemia agents crossing the placenta and stimulating the beta cell are rightly deemed inappropriate.

In the 1990s Langer and co-workers suggested that passage of glibenclamide (known in the US as glyburide) across the placenta was limited. Later they demonstrated that a treatment strategy starting glibenclamide was associated with similar birth outcomes to a strategy involving initial treatment with insulin in women with gestational diabetes (Langer et al., 2000).

In the original study only 4% of women assigned glibenclamide progressed to insulin during pregnancy. Since then multiple studies have shown the need for insulin in about 20% of patients initially treated with glibenclamide (Moore, 2007).

More recently Rowan et al (Rowan et al., 2008) demonstrated that treatment with metformin resulted in similar outcomes to initial insulin treatment in gestational diabetes—although 46% of women in the metformin limb required supplemental treatment with insulin. 751 women with gestational diabetes were randomized to either metformin or usual treatment with insulin therapy. The most important finding of the trial was that with a detailed protocol for glycaemic control, outcomes of women randomized to metformin or initial insulin were equivalent. The safety profile for mothers appeared to be good. Gastrointestinal side effects led to discontinuation of metformin in 1.9% of women and reduction in dose in 8.8%. The primary outcome—a composite of neonatal hypoglycaemia, respiratory distress, need for phototherapy, 5 minute Apgar score below 7 or preterm birth (before 37 weeks) were no different between the two treatment groups, being present in 32.0% of the metformin group and 32.2% of the insulin group. Secondary outcomes including birth weight, neonatal anthropometrics and rates of large for gestational age (>90th percentile) were also equivalent between the groups. Metformin appeared to have good patient acceptability with 76.6% of women suggesting that they would choose metformin in a subsequent pregnancy compared to 27.2% of those initially assigned to insulin—however 46% of women in the metformin group required supplemental insulin treatment to maintain glycaemic control. Importantly, metformin was associated with a lower weight gain between enrolment in the trial and 36 or 37 weeks of pregnancy (0.4 ± 2.9 kg in the metformin group vs. 2.0 ± 3.3 kg in the insulin group; $p < 0.001$) (Rowan et al., 2008).

Notably metformin does cross the placenta and this has led to safety concerns. Issues around the use of metformin in early pregnancy are discussed in Chapter 9. Rowan et al. have also undertaken a safety review with examination of children at age two years without any long term metabolic effects of metformin exposure in utero being apparent.

There is limited evidence with regard to which women might be selected for metformin or glibenclamide. For glibenclamide it is suggested from examination of the existing randomized control trial and observational series that failure of glibenclamide is more likely when initial fasting glucose is higher (above 6.4 mmol/l) (Moore, 2007). These observations make *a priori* sense as women with higher glucose levels are likely to have more severe disease. Similarly women presenting earlier in pregnancy would appear less suitable for oral agents. Similarly for metformin, women who required supplemental insulin had higher BMI in early pregnancy 33.6 ± 8.6 kg/m² vs. 31.1 ± 7.8 kg/m² than those maintained on metformin and higher baseline glucose levels (requiring supplemental insulin 6.1 ± 1.1 mmol/l, not requiring supplemental insulin 5.3 ± 0.8 mmol/l) (Rowan et al., 2008).

4.6 **Management of gestational diabetes: insulin**

Where dietary therapy fails insulin is instituted usually in a four or five times daily pattern, with short-acting insulin prior to meals and intermediate or long-acting insulin used once or twice daily. Short-acting insulin analogues have been examined in pregnancy with limited evidence of improved efficacy compared to traditional human insulin—essentially showing lower post-prandial peaks after administration. The ability to inject these insulins immediately before eating is an attractive feature.

For the long-acting analogues there is no randomized evidence suggesting benefit specifically in the context of gestational diabetes—issues around the safety and use of specific insulin regimens are discussed in Chapter 2.

Further reading

Bonomo M, Cetin I, Pisoni MP et al. (2004). Flexible treatment of gestational diabetes modulated on ultrasound evaluation of intrauterine growth: a controlled randomized clinical trial. *Diabetes Metab* **30**: 237–44.

Buchanan TA, Kjos SL, Montoro MN et al. (1994). Use of fetal ultrasound to select metabolic therapy for pregnancies complicated by mild gestational diabetes. *Diabetes Care* **17**: 275–83.

Crowther CA, Hiller JE, Moss JR et al. (2005). Effect of treatment of gestational diabetes mellitus on pregnancy outcomes. *New Engl J Med* **352**: 2477–2486.

de Veciana M, Major CA, Morgan MA, et al. (1995). Postprandial versus preprandial blood glucose monitoring in women with gestational diabetes mellitus requiring insulin therapy. *N Engl J Med* **333**: 1237–41.

HAPO Study Cooperative Research Group (2010). Hyperglycaemia and Adverse Pregnancy Outcome (HAPO) Study, associations with maternal body mass index. *BJOG* **117**: 575-84.

International Association of Diabetes and Pregnancy Study Groups Consensus Panel (2010). International Association of Diabetes and Pregnancy Study Groups recommendations on the diagnosis and classification of hyperglycemia in pregnancy. *Diabetes Care* **33**: 676–82.

Kjos SL, Schaefer-Graf U, Sardesi S, *et al.* (2001). A randomized controlled trial using glycemic plus fetal ultrasound parameters versus glycemic parameters to determine insulin therapy in gestational diabetes with fasting hyperglycemia. *Diabetes Care* **24**: 1904–10.

Landon MB, Spong CY, Thom E, *et al.* (2009). A multicenter, randomized trial of treatment for mild gestational diabetes. *N Engl J Med* **361**: 1339–48.

Langer O, Conway DL, Berkus MD, Xenakis EM, Gonzales O (2000). A comparison of glyburide and insulin in women with gestational diabetes mellitus. *N Engl J Med* **343**: 1134–8.

Metzger BE, Lowe LP, Dyer AR, *et al.* (2008). Hyperglycemia and adverse pregnancy outcomes. *N Engl J Med* **358**: 1991–2002.

Moore TR (2007). Glyburide for the treatment of gestational diabetes. A critical appraisal. *Diabetes Care* **30** Suppl 2: S209–13.

Rossi G, Somigliana E, Moschetta M (2000). Adequate timing of fetal ultrasound to guide metabolic therapy in mild gestational diabetes mellitus. Results from a randomized study. *Acta Obstet Gynecol Scand* **79**: 649–54.

Rowan JA, Hague WM, Gao W, Battin MR, Moore MP (2008). Metformin versus insulin for the treatment of gestational diabetes. *N Engl J Med* **358**: 2003–15.

Rowan JA, Gao W, Hague WM, McIntyre HD (2010). Glycemia and its relationship to outcomes in the metformin in gestational diabetes trial. *Diabetes Care* **33**: 9–16.

Schaefer-Graf UM, Kjos SL, Buhling KJ, *et al.* (2003). Amniotic fluid insulin levels and fetal abdominal circumference at time of amniocentesis in pregnancies with diabetes. *Diabet Med* **20**: 349–54.

Schaefer-Graf UM, Kjos SL, Fauzan OH, *et al.* (2004). A randomized trial evaluating a predominantly fetal growth-based strategy to guide management of gestational diabetes in Caucasian women. *Diabetes Care* **27**: 297–302.

Scott DA, Loveman E, McIntyre L, Waugh N (2002). Screening for gestational diabetes: a systematic review and economic evaluation. *Health Technol Assess* **6**: 1–161.

Yogev Y, Catalano PM (2009). Pregnancy and obesity. *Obstet Gynecol Clin North Am* **36**: 285–300, viii.

Chapter 5

Antenatal management of the diabetic pregnancy

Eleanor Jarvie and Scott M Nelson

Key points

- Pre-existing diabetes is associated with an increased risk of miscarriage, congenital abnormalities, intrauterine death, macrosomia, pre-term delivery (spontaneous and iatrogenic), shoulder dystocia, and perinatal morbidity and mortality.
- The incidence of congenital anomalies is directly related to maternal glycaemic control.
- Optimal detection of deviant fetal growth and macrosomia are by measurement of abdominal circumference.
- Shoulder dystocia is more frequent at lower birth weights in pregnancies complicated by maternal diabetes due to increased neonatal fat mass, but predictive models are poor.
- Induction of labour at 38 weeks is associated with a reduction in perinatal complications.

47

5.1 Introduction

The recent significant improvements in outcome of diabetic pregnancy are attributable to improved perinatal maternal glycaemic control, close antepartum surveillance, and advances in neonatal care. With appropriately treated gestational diabetes, the likelihood of fetal death is equivalent to background rates. In contrast currently pre-existing diabetes continue to have increased risk of adverse perinatal outcome. The complications include an increase in perinatal mortality, congenital malformations, deviated fetal growth (macrosomia and growth restriction), metabolic complications, birth trauma, and resultant increase in neonatal unit admissions. Ultrasound is the mainstay modality for monitoring diabetic pregnancies and potentially improving both perinatal management and fetal outcome. The timings and purpose of ultrasound are indicated in Table 5.1.

5.2 **Congenital anomalies**

Congenital anomalies have now replaced stillbirth and respiratory distress as the major cause of morbidity and mortality in infants of diabetic mothers. Their estimated frequency is 6–10%, or 3 to 5-fold higher than the general population, and is directly related to periconceptual and early pregnancy glycaemic control (Table 5.2). However, although there is a preponderance of cardiac and neural tube defects, diabetes is not associated with a specific fetal phenotype or syndrome, but rather affects multiple organ systems (Table 5.3). Detailed anomaly scans including visualization of the outflow tracts should be offered at 20 weeks gestation as the diagnostic accuracy is improved at this later gestation. Chromosomal abnormalities have equivalent prevalence in diabetic pregnancy and screening should be offered in the same manner as routine care.

5.3 **Growth abnormalities**

Fetal macrosomia complicates approximately a third of pregnancies in women with established diabetes mellitus and 25% of pregnancies affected by gestational diabetes mellitus (GDM). In women with established vascular disease, or those that develop hypertensive complications, intrauterine growth restriction (IUGR) may develop. Consequently estimation of fetal growth and amniotic fluid volume are recommended to be undertaken at 28, 32, 36, and 38 weeks. For those women wishing to continue the pregnancy, weekly monitoring would then be instigated. Although serial measurements of abdominal circumference (AC) and femur length (FL) are conventionally plotted, an absolute AC rather than growth velocity is still the best predictor of birthweight including small for gestational age (<10th centile) and macrosomia (>4 kg). However, accelerated and declining fetal growth have been linked to increased risk of fetal mortality hence prompting earlier intervention. An additional novel role for the estimation of fetal growth has been recently developed in gestational diabetes where there are now several studies incorporating ultrasound and estimates of fetal weight to direct insulin therapy.

Table 5.1 Use of ultrasound during pregnancy

Scan	Type of USS	Purpose of scan	What is measured?	Potential diabetic complication
Early scan	Prior to 10 weeks (transabdominal or transvaginal)	Confirm continuing pregnancy	Number of embryos, crown rump length 6–13 weeks	Miscarriage
Dating scan	10+0 – 13+6 weeks	Gestational age assessment	Heart beat visualized, crown rump length (6–13 weeks), head circumference and femur length (13–25 weeks)	Major neural tube defects
Nuchal translucency scan	11+0 – 14+6 weeks	Screening modality for chromosomal abnormalities e.g. Down syndrome	Nuchal fold	No specific increased risk of chromosomal defects
Detailed anomaly scan	18+0 – 20+6 weeks	Assessment of fetal anatomy	Head and neck (skull, brain, cavum pellicidum, ventricular atrium cerebellum), face (lips), chest (four chamber cardiac views, outflow tracts and lungs), abdomen (stomach, short portion of intra-hepatic section of the umbilical vein, abdominal wall, bowel, renal pelvis, bladder), spine (vertebrae and skin covering), limbs (femur, metacarpals, metatarsals). Measurements include head circumference, measurement of lateral ventricle, sub-occipital-bregmatic diameter, abdominal circumference and femur length	Neural tube defects Skeletal abnormalities Sacral agenesis (rare) Cardiac septal and outflow tract malformations
Growth scans	From 21 weeks, repeated 4 weekly From 36 weeks, Repeated 2 weekly	Assessment of amniotic fluid volume and fetal growth. Umbilical Doppler assessment in high risk patients	Head circumference, abdominal circumference, femur length, liquor volume.	Polyhydramnios Macrosomia Growth restriction Placental vasculopathy

Table 5.2 Derived absolute risk of a major or minor congenital anomaly in association with the number of standard deviations (SD) of glycosylated haemoglobin above normal. and the approximate corresponding HbA_{1c} concentration, measured periconceptionally

SD of GHb	Corresponding HbA_{1c} (%)	Corresponding HbA_{1c} (nmol/mol)	Absolute risk of a congenital anomaly (%, 95% CI)
0	5.0	31	2.2 (0.0 to 4.4)
2	6.0	42	3.2 (0.4 to 6.1)
4	7.0	53	4.8 (1.0 to 8.6)
6	8.0	64	7.0 (1.7 to 12.3)
8	9.0	75	10.1 (2.3 to 17.8)
10	10.0	86	14.4 (2.8 to 25.9)
≥12	≥11	≥97	20.1 (3.0 to 37.1)

Assumes a DCCT-aligned HbA_{1c} assay with mean (SD) of 5.0% (0.5%) among non-diabetic, non-pregnant controls. From Guerin A et al. (2007) Diabetes Care **30**: 1920–5.

With respect to sonographic umbilical Doppler studies in patients with pregnancies complicated by pre-existing hypertensive disease, IUGR and vasculopathy, their use can reduce adverse outcomes. However, at present there are no firm guidelines regarding the use of this tool for routine surveillance in diabetic pregnancies although it is accepted as being a better tool of fetal wellbeing than fetal cardiotocography or biophysical profile.

5.4 Cardiotocography

Antenatal cardiotocography (CTG), although classically used to assess fetal wellbeing, has not been shown to have a significant effect on perinatal morbidity or mortality. However, the four trials which have been undertaken—although including intermediate and high risk women—only had in total 1,588 women and therefore are substantially underpowered to detect a difference in stillbirth. As a consequence of this CTG continues to be used routinely although the optimum frequency of testing is unclear as once a week testing is insufficient to reduce perinatal mortality, despite NICE recommending weekly monitoring of fetal wellbeing after 38 weeks' gestation. In contrast during labour there is a clear role for continuous CTG monitoring as maternal hyperglycaemia has been associated with fetal distress and diabetic pregnancies have an increased risk of need for operative delivery.

Table 5.3 Congenital abnormalities associated with pre-existing diabetes mellitus	
Organ system	**Details of abnormalities**
Cardiac abnormalities	Transposition of great vessels Ventricular septal defects Coarctation of aorta Atrial septal defects Cardiomyopathy
Skeletal	Vertebral & rib defects Limb reduction defects Scaral agenesis (rare but classical defect of diabetic pregnancy)
Central nervous system	Anencephaly Neural tube defect Microcephaly Hydrocephalus
Uro-genital system	Hydronephrosis Renal agenesis Ureteral duplication Multicystic dysplasia Hydrospadias
Gastrointestinal tract	Duodenal atresia Ano-rectal atresia Oesophageal atresia
Facial	Cleft lip and palate Ear malformations (microtia, anotia, ear canal atresia, hearing loss) Eye anomalies (cataract, coloboma, optic nerve hypoplasia)

5.5 **Timing and mode of delivery**

Several studies have examined the optimal timing of birth in women with diabetes. Notably routine induction of labour at 38 weeks' gestation reduces the incidence of large for gestational age babies and shoulder dystocia, but not at the cost of an increased caesarean section rate. More recent studies examining routine induction for pregnancy induced hypertension at 36 weeks' gestation have also not shown increases in caesarean section. Given that the risk of respiratory complications in the newborn are directly related to gestational age at birth and diabetes further increases this risk, many units are now considering use of corticosteroids even at this late stage in pregnancy. Corticosteroids significantly reduce the risk of transient

Table 5.4 Programme of obstetric monitoring for women with diabetes, derived from current NICE and SIGN guidelines

Appointment	Care for women with diabetes during pregnancy	Additional points
First appointment – pre-pregnancy counselling (joint diabetes and antenatal care)	• Offer information, advice and support in relation to optimizing glycaemic control. • Take a clinical history to establish the extent of diabetic-related complications. • Review medications for diabetes and its complications. • Offer retinal and/or renal assessment if these have not been undertaken in the previous 12 months.	Maternal U&Es, MSSU, microalbuminaemia HbA$_{1C}$
7–9 weeks	Confirm viability of pregnancy and gestational age by ultrasound	
Booking appointment (ideally by 10 weeks)	Discuss information, education and advice on how DM will affect pregnancy, birth and early parenting (breastfeeding)	First trimester screening
16 weeks	Offer retinal assessment at 16–20 weeks to women with pre-existing DM who have shown signs of diabetic retinopathy at their first antenatal appointment	Offer routine second trimester screening
20 weeks	Offer routine details anomaly scanning with four chamber view of the heart and the outflow tracts	
28 weeks	Offer ultrasound monitoring for fetal growth and amniotic fluid volume. Offer retinal assessment to those women with no previous signs of diabetic retinopathy	
32 weeks	Offer ultrasound monitoring for fetal growth and amniotic fluid volume	Offer investigations that would be part routine care

36 weeks	Offer ultrasound monitoring for fetal growth and amniotic fluid volume.
	Offer information and advice about:
	• Timing and, mode and management of delivery.
	• Analgesia and anaesthesia.
	• Changes in hypoglycaemic therapy during and after childbirth.
	• Management of the baby at birth.
	✗ • Initiation of breast feeding and the effect of breast feeding on glycaemic control. ✗
	• Contraception and follow up. by G.P.
38 weeks	Offer induction of labour, or caesarean section if indicated, and start regular tests of fetal wellbeing for women with diabetes who are awaiting spontaneous labour (CTG, fetal growth, liquor volume, umbilical artery Doppler)
39 weeks	Offer tests for fetal wellbeing (CTG, fetal growth, liquor volume, umbilical artery Doppler)
40 weeks	Offer tests for fetal wellbeing (CTG, fetal growth, liquor volume, umbilical artery Doppler)
41 weeks	Offer tests for fetal wellbeing (CTG, fetal growth, liquor volume, umbilical artery Doppler)

tachypnoea of the newborn and respiratory distress syndrome even if administered at 37 weeks' gestation, and although corticosteroids can induce maternal hyperglycaemia, this can often be managed by planned increases in insulin.

The mode of delivery in the diabetic patient is best decided on an individual basis with input from the patient, diabetologist and obstetrician as diabetes itself is not an indication for caesarean section. Instead elective caesarean section is often considered for large babies and indeed is recommended for diabetics with an estimated fetal weight >4.5 kg, as it removes the risk of shoulder dystocia at vaginal delivery and the subsequent risk of nerve injury and birth asphyxia. With respect to women who wish to consider vaginal birth after caesarean section, birthweight is the primary determinant of success and women with diabetes are less likely to be successful than the normal population which have a 70% chance of achieving a vaginal birth. For women who have had a previous delivery complicated by shoulder dystocia, elective caesarean delivery is appropriate.

5.6 **Conclusion**

Although broadly empirical, enhanced antenatal surveillance (Table 5.4) must consist of close maternal and fetal monitoring with the aim of identifying additional risk factors and the early signs of fetal and maternal compromise.

Further reading

Coomarasamy A, Connock M, Thornton J, Khan KS (2005). Accuracy of ultrasound biometry in the prediction of macrosomia: a systematic quantitative review. *BJOG* **112** (11): 1461–6.

Graves CRM (2007). Antepartum fetal surveillance and timing of delivery in the pregnancy complicated by diabetes mellitus. *Clinical Obstetrics & Gynecology* **50**: 1007–13.

Massi-Benedetti M, Federici MO, Di Renzo GC (2008). Management of gestational diabetes mellitus. In Hod M, Jovanovic L, Di Renzo GC, De Leiva A & Langer O (Eds). *Textbook of Diabetes and Pregnancy*, 2nd ed. Informa Healthcare, London.

Nizard J, Ville Y (2009). The fetus of a diabetic mother: sonographic evaluation. *Seminars in Fetal and Neonatal Medicine* **14**: 101–5.

National Institute for Health and Clinical Excellence (2008). *Clinical guideline 62: Antenatal care: routine care for the healthy pregnant woman.* NICE, London.

National Institute for Health and Clinical Excellence (2008). *Clinical guideline 63: Diabetes in pregnancy management of diabetes and its complications from pre-conception to the postnatal period.* NICE, London.

Royal College of Obstetricians and Gynaecologists (Revised 2004). Antenatal corticosteroids to prevent respiratory distress syndrome (Green-top 7). RCOG, London. http://www.rcog.org.uk/womens-health/clinical-guidance/antenatal-corticosteroids-prevent-respiratory-distress-syndrome-gree

Royal College of Obstetricians and Gynaecologists (2005). Shoulder dystocia (Green-top 42). RCOG, London. http://www.rcog.org.uk/womens-health/clinical-guidance/shoulder-dystocia-green-top-42

Stutchfield P, Whitaker R, Russell I; Antenatal Steroids for Term Elective Caesarean Section (ASTECS) Research Team (2005). Antenatal betamethasone and incidence of neonatal respiratory distress after elective caesarean section: pragmatic randomised trial. *BMJ* **331**: 662.

Suhonen L, Hiilesmaa V, Teramo K (2000). Glycaemic control during early pregnancy and fetal malformations in women with type I diabetes mellitus. *Diabetologia* **43**: 79–82.

Chapter 6

Diabetes management during labour

Rosemary Temple

Key points

- Preparation of women for birth should include education about the increased metabolic stresses of labour and how blood glucose will be controlled during labour and birth
- Maternal hyperglycaemia during labour increases the risk of neonatal hypoglycaemia
- High levels of stress hormones released during labour increase risk of maternal hyperglycaemia
- Insulin requirements fall immediately following birth of the baby.

6.1 Introduction

6.1.1 Preparation of the woman for labour

The birth of a baby is a stressful time for any woman. However, for the woman with pre-gestational diabetes (PGDM) or gestational diabetes (GDM), there are additional challenges, including timing and mode of delivery and how best to achieve excellent blood glucose levels throughout labour and delivery. The woman has usually been encouraged to self-manage her blood glucose throughout the pregnancy and may find it difficult to hand over her glucose control during labour to healthcare professionals.

It is important to discuss what may happen at the time of the birth with the woman and her partner so they are well prepared. This discussion includes choices for pain relief, advice on breastfeeding, an explanation of possible neonatal problems, the importance of good blood glucose control during labour and how this will be achieved.

Women should be encouraged to write a 'birth wish list' but also advised why it may not be possible to follow all requests on this list.

6.1.2 **Risks for development of neonatal hypoglycaemia**

Risk of neonatal hypoglycaemia is increased for two reasons. Firstly, poor maternal glycaemic control during later pregnancy leads to chronic fetal hyperinsulinism as a response to the mother's high glucose levels crossing the placenta and increases risk of neonatal hypoglycaemia. Secondly, maternal hyperglycaemia during labour leads to fetal hyperinsulinism and subsequent neonatal hypoglycaemia in the early hours following birth.

Several observational studies have shown maternal hyperglycemia during labour increases risk of neonatal hypoglycaemia (Table 6.1). One recent study, of 107 women with type 1 diabetes, showed neonatal blood glucose was usually below 2.5 mmol/l if maternal blood glucose was above 8 mmol/l during labour (Taylor, 2002).

6.2 **Glucose management during labour and delivery**

During labour and birth, blood glucose should be measured hourly and maintained between 4 and 7 mmol/l, using an intravenous insulin infusion if necessary.

6.2.1 **Labour and delivery in women with pregestational diabetes (type 1 and 2)**

Women should eat normally and have their usual insulin regime until they are in active labour (3 cm dilated or undergoing amniotomy). Women

Table 6.1 Studies of maternal blood glucose during labour and risk of neonatal hypoglycaemia

Author	Year	Number	Type of DM	Results
Anderson	1983	53	T1	Negative correlation between maternal BG and fetal BG, $r = -0.46$, $p < 0.001$)
Miodovnik	1987	122	T1	47% babies hypo if maternal BG > 5 mmol/l vs 14% if maternal BG < 5 mmol/l
Curet	1997	233	T1 & T2	Maternal BG lower if no neonatal hypoglycaemia
Lean	1990	25	Insulin treated	Negative correlation between maternal BG and fetal BG, $r = -0.58$, $p = 0.01$
Balsells	2000	85	GDM	Maternal BG in last 2 hrs of labour associated with neonatal hypoglycaemia
Taylor	2002	107	T1	Negative correlation between maternal BG and fetal BG, $r = -0.33$, $p < 0.001$

Table 6.2 Insulin infusion regime for women during active labour (see text)

Total daily insulin dose	<40 units	40–59 units	60–89 units	>90 units
Blood glucose mmol/l	Insulin u/hour	Insulin u/hour	Insulin u/hour	Insulin u/hour
0–3	0	0	0	0
3.1–6.9	1.0	1.5	2.0	2.0
7.0–8.9	1.5	2.0	3.0	4.0
9.0–10.9	2.0	3.0	4.0	5.0
11.0–15.0	3.0	4.0	5.0	6.0
>15.0	Call doctor	Call doctor	Call doctor	Call doctor

using insulin glargine or insulin detemir as their basal insulin should continue with this but short-acting and intermediate-acting insulins should be discontinued and an intravenous insulin regime commenced.

A syringe pump is set up with 50 units insulin in 50 ml normal saline and 5% dextrose solution containing 20 mmol/l potassium chloride per litre is commenced at 100 ml per hour. Blood glucose is measured hourly. It is important to use an insulin infusion scale related to both insulin requirements in late pregnancy and the blood glucose level (Table 6.2). If the woman has two consecutive readings above 9 mmol/l, the insulin sliding scale is changed to the column on the right so a higher insulin scale is used to achieve normoglycaemia. If the woman has two glucose values below 4 mmol/l, the scale is shifted to the column on the left.

This regime is particularly useful now there are many women with obesity and insulin resistance.

Following delivery, the insulin infusion rate should be reduced to the lowest scale (i.e. on far left of Table 6.2) and blood glucose should be monitored hourly until the woman is eating and can return to her usual insulin regime.

6.2.2 **Elective caesarean section**

Women with diabetes should be put as the second case on a morning list and an insulin infusion set up at 6 am (Table 6.2). In addition blood glucose should be checked during the night and insulin infusion commenced earlier if blood glucose levels are unstable.

6.3 **Glucose management in women with gestational diabetes**

Blood glucose should be monitored hourly in all women with GDM throughout active labour or if having delivery by caesarean section.

If blood glucose rises above 7 mmol/l on two occasions, an intravenous insulin regime should be commenced (Table 6.2). Women with GDM are often overweight and insulin resistant so healthcare professionals need to be aware that women may rapidly need to shift to a higher insulin scale. Recent research has confirmed that this approach of watchful management in women with GDM is usually successful and avoids the need for routine insulin infusion (Barrett, 2009). For management of women with pre-gestational diabetes, see Figure 6.1.

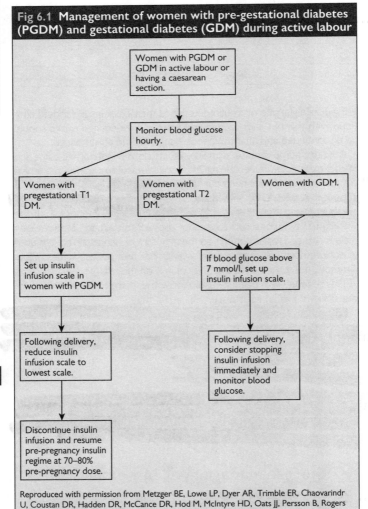

Fig 6.1 **Management of women with pre-gestational diabetes (PGDM) and gestational diabetes (GDM) during active labour**

Reproduced with permission from Metzger BE, Lowe LP, Dyer AR, Trimble ER, Chaovarindr U, Coustan DR, Hadden DR, McCance DR, Hod M, McIntyre HD, Oats JJ, Persson B, Rogers MS and Sacks DA: Hyperglycemia and adverse pregnancy outcomes. *N Engl J Med* **358**:1991-2002, 2008.

6.4 **Conclusion**

Risk of neonatal hypoglycaemia is related to maternal glucose levels during labour and delivery, and therefore tight maternal blood glucose control is essential. All women with diabetes should be advised of this before labour so they are well prepared for the extra care they may need to achieve this.

Further reading

Andersen O, Hertel J, Schmølker L, Kühl C, et al. (1985). Influence of the maternal plasma glucose concentration at delivery on the risk of hypoglycaemia in infants of insulin dependent mothers. *Acta Paediatrica Scandinavica* **74**: 268–73.

Balsells M, Corcoy R, Adelantado JM, Garc′a-Patterson A, Altirriba O, de Leiva A (2000). Gestational diabetes: metabolic control during labour. *Diabetes Nutr Metab* **13**: 257–62.

Barrett HL, Morris J, McElduff A (2009). Watchful waiting: a management protocol for maternal glycaemia in the peripartum period. *Aust NZ J Obstet Gynaecol* **49**: 162–7.

Curet LB, Izquierdo LA, Gilson GJ, et al. (1997). Relative effects of antepartum and intrapartum maternal blood glucose levels on incidence of neonatal hypoglycaemia. *Journal of Perinataology* **17**: 113–5.

Lean ME, Pearson DW, Sutherland HW (1990). Insulin management during labour and delivery in mothers with diabetes. *Diabetic Medicine* **7**: 162–4.

Miodovnik M, Mimouni F, Tsang RC (1987). Management of the insulin-dependent diabetic during labour and delivery. Influences on neonatal outcome. *American Journal of Perinataology* **4**: 106–14.

Taylor R, Lee C, Kyne-Grzebalski D, et al. (2002). Clinical outcomes of pregnancy in women with type 1 diabetes. *Obstet Gynecol* **99**: 537–41.

Chapter 7

Infant of diabetic mother

Lesley Jackson and Robert Lindsay

> **Key Points**
>
> - Strict maternal pre-pregnancy glycaemic control reduces the incidence of fetal malformations and anomalies in pregnancies complicated by diabetes
> - Tight maternal glycaemic control during labour and delivery may reduce neonatal hypoglycaemia
> - Current fetal monitoring techniques cannot reliably detect fetal compromise which may lead to premature delivery which can compound neonatal morbidity.

7.1 Introduction

Diabetes mellitus, whether pre-existing or gestational, is the commonest maternal medical condition to complicate pregnancy (HAPO, 2002). Glucose intolerance during human pregnancy can adversely affect the intrauterine environment, impacting upon the fetus and neonate with a variety of adverse outcomes described (Table 7.1) (Penney et al., 2003). This chapter will focus upon the effects of maternal diabetes upon the infant of the diabetic mother (IDM).

7.2 Congenital anomalies

Despite major improvements in the care of pregnant women with diabetes, the three-to-five fold increased incidence in congenital anomalies relative to the general population has shown little temporal change (Table 7.2) (Reece et al., 1998; Wren et al., 2003). A linear relationship between glycosylated haemoglobin (HbA$_{1c}$) concentrations and malformation rates has been reported, with poor glycaemic control in the pre- and early post-conception period being critical to subsequent malformation risk (Ylinen et al., 1984; Miller et al., 1981; Baker et al., 1981).

Table 7.1 Adverse outcomes in offspring of mothers with type 1 diabetes	
Biochemical	**Growth and development**
Hypocalcaemia	Congenital anomalies
Polycythaemia and hyperviscosity	Fetal overgrowth
Hyperbilirubinaemia	Increased adiposity
Hypoglycaemia/hyperinsulinaemia	Growth restriction
	Hypertrophic cardiomyopathy
Diseases of prematurity	**Mortality**
Respiratory distress syndrome	Increased perinatal mortality: stillbirth and neonatal death
Transient tachypnoea of the newborn	

During the period of organogenesis, prior to the seventh week of gestation, the diabetic intrauterine environment appears crucial. Unfortunately, most anomalies occur before pregnancy is recognized, highlighting the need for optimal maternal pre-conception glycaemic control. The aetiology of diabetic embryopathy is not fully elucidated. Theories suggest a complex interplay between maternal hyperglycaemia and fetal fuel metabolism, with resultant disruption of cellular signalling and genotoxic effects. Hyperglycaemia increases the concentration of free oxygen radicals and also alters yolk sac differentiation, a developmental step disrupted by multiple teratogens (Reece et al., 1994). Hypoglycaemia has also been associated with congenital malformations in animal models but human corroborative data are lacking. The possibility therefore remains that extremes of glycaemic control may promote teratogenesis in human pregnancy.

IDMs are at risk of a wide variety of malformations, those most frequently reported are summarized in Table 7.2.

7.3 Macrosomia

Macrosomia, defined as a birthweight exceeding the 90th centile for gestation or birthweight exceeding absolute values of 4 or 4.5 kg, commonly complicates diabetic pregnancy, with 35% to 70% of IDMs having birth weight >90th percentile. Macrosomia is related to increased adiposity and tissue-specific organomegaly, affecting the liver and myocardium in particular. Skeletal length is increased in proportion to weight, whereas brain size is not increased such that

Table 7.2 Congenital anomalies frequently observed in infants of diabetic mothers

Cardiovascular
Congenital heart disease including ventricular septal defect and transposition of the great vessels (8.5 per 100 live births)

Skeletal
Caudal regression sequence (agenesis or hypoplasia of the femora occurs in conjunction with agenesis of the lower vertebrae, relative risk in IDMs of 212 compared with non-diabetics)
Sacral agenesis
Vertebral dysplasia

Central nervous system
(5.3 per 100 live births)
Anencephaly
Meningomyelocele and spina bifida

Gastrointestinal
Small left colon syndrome (an abnormality that is unique to IDMs, a transient inability to pass meconium that resolves spontaneously)

head circumference may appear disproportionally small in relative to the remainder of the body. Such infants are often described as being 'cherub-like', their increased size also being associated with facial plethora — *excessive red blood cell production*

Macrosomia is thought to result from fetal hyperinsulinaemia, which characterizes many diabetic pregnancies: maternal hyperglycaemia promotes insulin secretion from the fetal pancreas, as evidenced by increased umbilical cord insulin and c-peptide concentrations, the anabolic effects of which stimulate protein, lipid and glycogen synthesis promoting organomegaly and macrosomia (Lepercq et al., 2001).

Although conflicting associations have been reported, the consensus of available evidence does not support a simple relationship between overall maternal glycaemic control and resultant macrosomia. Consensus has also not been reached on whether strict maternal glycaemic control, either early or late in pregnancy, could have the most effect on reducing the incidence of macrosomia, although it is known that increased abdominal circumference, a surrogate for weight gain and eventual macrosomia, can be observed from 24 weeks of gestation in pregnant women with diabetes (Jovanic-Peterson et al., 1991, Stott et al., 2004).

The macrosomic fetus may cause obstetric concern in later pregnancy. Increased risks of shoulder dystocia, obstructed labour, instrumented delivery and caesarean section with the potential for subsequent intrapartum compromise are well described. Birth trauma, including brachial plexus injuries and similar nerve palsies, are also more frequent in macrosomic infants.

7.4 Intra-uterine growth restriction

Although less common than macrosomia, a proportion of IDMs grow poorly during pregnancy, as a consequence of placental insufficiency, which can result in intrauterine growth restriction (IUGR), defined as a gestation-corrected birthweight of < 2nd centile. Placental insufficiency and IUGR are more prevalent in women who have pre-established microvascular complications of diabetes, most notably diabetic nephropathy. This group of infants have an increased risk of hypoglycaemia in the early days of life and may also be at greater risk of cardiovascular morbidity in adulthood related to adverse metabolic programming consequent upon intrauterine malnutrition.

serious kidney-related complication.

7.5 Respiratory complications

high resp

Within the first day of life many IDMs become tachypnoeic, defined as a respiratory rate >60 breaths/minute. The differential diagnosis is wide but frequently related to transient tachypnoea of the newborn (TTN) and the relative surfactant deficiency of respiratory distress syndrome (RDS). Hypoglycaemia, hypothermia, polycythaemia, cardiac failure and cerebral irritation resulting from traumatic delivery all require consideration.

high resps for 48 hrs.

To reduce the recognized risk of late intra-uterine death, IDMs are frequently electively delivered at 37–38 weeks' gestation. Such elective deliveries, particularly by caesarean section, do not prepare the fetus for independent breathing as the labour-induced stress hormone surge that initiates pulmonary fluid absorption does not occur. Consequently, fetal pulmonary fluid clearance is delayed and TTN is more prevalent. Obstetricians carefully plan elective deliveries to balance the risks of late intra-uterine death and early neonatal respiratory compromise, prescribing exogenous antenatal glucocorticoids to promote fetal lung maturation when delivery is planned prior to 38 completed weeks.

RDS is more common in IDMs relative to gestation-matched infants of non-diabetic mothers (Robert et al., 1976). It has been suggested that the increased incidence of RDS relates to the opposing effects that insulin and cortisol have on pulmonary surfactant synthesis: insulin inhibits surfactant synthesis by type 2 pneumocytes whereas cortisol promotes surfactant synthesis, hence the antenatal use of fluorinated glucocorticoid to promote fetal lung maturation when prematurity threatens.

7.6 Hypocalcaemia

Neonatal hypocalcaemia, defined as a corrected calcium concentration of < 1.7 mmol/l, has been reported in up to 50% of IDMs and is related to maternal glycaemic control in late pregnancy (Mimouni et al., 1986). When present, hypocalcaemia is usually associated with hyperphosphataemia reflecting transient neonatal hypoparathyroidism, presumed to relate to maternal magnesium loss, which functionally inhibits parathyroid hormone release. Clinically this may present as transient jitteriness in the infant, though the frequent association with hypoglycaemia seen in these infants makes direct causation problematic. The lowest serum calcium concentration typically occurs between 24 to 72 hours after birth and usually resolves without treatment.

7.7 Polycythaemia and jaundice

IDMs have an increased incidence of polycythaemia, defined as a haematocrit >0.70, and as a consequence are more likely to develop neonatal hyperviscosity syndrome than healthy term infants (Mimouni et al., 1986). Neonatal hyperviscosity syndrome predisposes to thromboses, most notably of the renal vein and cerebral venous sinuses as well as other sites, which if present is associated with significant morbidity and increased mortality. Elevated umbilical erythropoietin concentrations have been reported in IDMs, the concentration correlated with fetal plasma insulin concentration. The elevated EPO concentrations observed in the IDM fetus and newborn reflect chronic hyperinsulinaemia which increases cellular glucose uptake and metabolic rate which produces relative cellular hypoxia.

Jaundice, reflecting unconjugated hyperbilirubinaemia, occurs frequently in IDMs in whom a longer clinical course in is anticipated consequent upon the lysis of a relatively increased red cell load, and perhaps also due to liver enzyme immaturity related to hyperinsulinaemia (Peevy et al., 1980). The jaundice responds well to phototherapy.

7.8 Hypertrophic cardiomyopathy

Cardiomegaly and hypertrophy were first described as being more frequent in IDMs in the 1940s. With improved echocardiology techniques the understanding of this condition has advanced. Generalized myocardial hypertrophy is the norm with disproportionate thickening of the ventricular septum. Severe hypertrophy with intermittent occlusion of the left ventricular outflow tract is required before clinical sequelae, which can result in intrauterine or neonatal death. Severity is related in part to maternal glycaemia control and fetal hyperinsulinaemia (Ullmo et al., 2007). The hypertrophic cardiomyopathy that occurs in IDMs is transient: symptoms usually resolve by 4 weeks with complete regression ventricular septal hypertrophy by 12 months or earlier without later-life sequelae (Way et al., 1979).

7.9 Hypoglycaemia

The definition of neonatal hypoglycaemia has been controversial, although most clinicians would currently define neonatal hypoglycaemia as a blood glucose concentration <2.6 mmol/l. Hypoglycaemia occurs considerably more frequently in IDMs, in one large series it was reported in 27% of infants (Cordero et al., 1988). The expected standard of care for such infants, whether cared for with their mothers on postnatal wards or in a neonatal unit, is to monitor for hypoglycaemia by following an established screening protocol using an approved near-patient testing device. Staff caring for such infants must be aware of the need for close observation and prompt treatment if hypoglycaemia ensues, with intensification of post-natal care and medical review when hypoglycaemia is recurrent. In most IDMs, hypoglycaemia is observed most frequently between 4 to 6 hours of age but can persist in excess of 48 hours after birth.

Depending on symptoms and severity, hypoglycaemia can be treated enterally, with increased milk volumes, or intravenously using dextrose solutions. Breast milk is the preferred milk, with standard term formula offered when not available. Premature or other higher calorie milks are not indicated for the treatment of hypoglycaemia in IDMs. Excessive boluses of intravenous dextrose should also be avoided to minimize continual stimulation and secretion of insulin by the neonatal pancreas.

The pathogenesis of the increased risk of hypoglycaemia observed in IDMs is multifactorial (Hawdon & Aynsley-Green, 1996). Maternal hyperglycaemia chronically activates the fetal pancreas with resultant β-cell hyperplasia and hyperinsulinaemia. At delivery the switch necessary to initiate independent endogenous glucose production is impaired by continuing hyperinsulinaemia in the newborn which predisposes to hypoglycaemia. IDMs are additionally vulnerable as the anabolic effects of hyperinsulinaemia prevent the utilization of alternative fat and protein substrates for metabolism, particularly ketone bodies which the neonatal brain can utilize. In addition, defective hormonal counter-regulation has also been implicated in the pathogenesis of hyopoglycaemia in IDM: plasma glucagon concentrations in IDMs after birth demonstrate a blunted response to hypoglycaemia relative to that observed in healthy term infants (Artal et al., 1982, Cowett et al., 1983).

7.10 Intrauterine death

The stillbirth rate in established diabetes remains five times that of the general population despite the intensive medical supervision such pregnancies receive (Casson et al., 1997). Late intrauterine death is more likely in poorly controlled diabetes and in macrosomic fetuses, but can complicate any diabetic pregnancy (Lauenborg et al., 2003). The pathophysiology of late intrauterine death is little understood (Siddiqui & James, 2003). Placental vascular insufficiency, most prevalent in women with pre-existing microvascular complications, is a well recognized risk factor which can be serially evaluated through ultrasonography. Maternal diabetes is a ketosis-prone condition. Ketosis reduces uterine blood flow and infusing ketones produces fetal hypoxia in animal models. As fetal hyperinsulinaemia increases cellular oxygen demand and consumption, episodic exposure to ketosis may augment the vulnerability of the IDM to this insult.

7.11 Long-term effects

The later life effects of in utero exposure to abnormal glucose metabolism as a result of maternal hyperglycaemia are now being investigated. It has long been suggested that infants of lower birth weight have an increased risk of certain metabolic abnormalities including most notably hypertension, type 2 diabetes and resultant cardiovascular disease (the Barker Hypothesis). In contrast to this an increase in the risk of obesity and type 2 diabetes is also suggested after in utero exposure to maternal diabetes. In a similar fashion to the explanation behind the Barker hypothesis it is suggested that the adverse intra-uterine environment experienced by the IDM result in fetal "programming" that is permanent alteration in function as a result of early environmental exposure.

Some of the earliest evidence of this came from studies in the Pima Indians—a native American group at high risk of obesity and type 2 diabetes. It was observed that offspring of mothers with diabetes were more likely than offspring of diabetic fathers to themselves develop obesity (Pettit et al., 1983) and type 2 diabetes (Pettit et al., 1988). This was of particular importance in the Pima population as the early onset of diabetes in mothers in this population resulted in high numbers of children and young adults developing type 2 diabetes. This in turn prompted Pettit to describe the "vicious cycle" of maternal diabetes where early onset diabetes in mothers in the Pima population resulted in earlier diabetes in their children and increasing prevalence of diabetes through the population. While a variety of explanations for the phenomenon observed in the Pima are possible—including shared environmental effects after birth or inheritance of mitochondrial genetic mutations—the most convincing explanation arising from the Pima group is that early environmental exposure to maternal diabetes in utero adds to an inherently high genetic risk of type 2 diabetes and obesity (Dabelea et al., 2000).

Since this work it has been observed that penetrance of some autosomal dominant forms of diabetes—the subtype of maturity onset diabetes of the young (MODY) caused by hepatocyte nuclear factor 1 alpha mutation—is also increased where mutations are inherited from mother rather than father (Stride et al., 2002). Since this is not an imprinted gene again the interpretation is that penetrance has been affected by the intrauterine environment.

For diabetes more generally this creates pressing questions as to whether the maternal environment is contributing to risk of diabetes and obesity in the offspring of mothers with type 1, type 2, and gestational diabetes. All of these conditions are potentially associated with fetal overgrowth. Recent studies have supported an increase in obesity and impaired glucose tolerance in offspring of mothers with type 1 diabetes. The study with the longest follow up examining offspring of mothers with type 1 diabetes in their early 20s showed an increase in "pre diabetes" (impaired fasting glucose and impaired glucose tolerance) (Clausen et al., 2009). It appears therefore that there is a similar increase in risk of obesity and at least some impairment in glucose tolerance in infants of mothers with type 1 diabetes. Mothers with gestational diabetes have, on average, a more modest increase in glucose levels during pregnancy. Conversely the far greater numbers (ranging between 2 and 20% of deliveries depending on diagnostic criteria and risk factors in the population) mean that any such programming effects would have a far greater public health importance. At present the programming role of gestational diabetes and indeed whether there are additional effects of maternal obesity to programme offspring metabolic disease remain unclear.

Further reading

Artal R, Platt LD, Kammula RK (1982). Sympathoadrenal activity in infants of diabetic mothers. *Am J Obstet Gynecol* **142**: 436–9.

Baker L, Egler J, Klein S, Goldman A (1981). Meticulous control of diabetes during pregnancy prevents congenital lumosacral defects in rats. *Diabetes* **30**: 955–9.

Casson IF, Clarke CA, Howard CV, Pennycook S, Pharoah POD, Walkinshaw S (1997). Outcomes of pregnancy in insulin dependent diabetic women: results of a five year population cohort study. *BMJ* **35**: 275–8.

Clausen TD, Mathiesen ER, Hansen T, Pedersen O, Jensen DM, Lauenborg J, Damm P (2008). High prevalence of type 2 diabetes and pre-diabetes in adult offspring of women with gestational diabetes mellitus or type 1 diabetes: the role of intrauterine hyperglycemia. *Diabetes Care* **31**: 340–6.

Cordero L, Treuer SH, Landon MB, Gabbe SG (1988). Management of infants of diabetic mothers. *Arch Paediatr Adolesc Med* **152**: 249–53.

Cowett RM, Susa JB, Giletti B (1983). Glucose kinetics in infants of diabetic mothers. *Am J Obstet Gynecol* **146**: 781–6.

Dabelea D, Hanson RL, Lindsay RS, et al. (2000). Intrauterine exposure to diabetes conveys risks for type 2 diabetes and obesity: a study of discordant sibships. *Diabetes* **49**: 2208–11.

HAPO Study Cooperative Research Group (2008). Hyperglycemia and adverse pregnancy outcomes. *N Engl J Med* **358**: 1991–2002.

Hawdon JM, Aynsley-Green A (1996). Neonatal complications including hypoglycaemia. In: Dornhorst A, Hadden D (Eds). *Diabetes and Pregnancy: an international approach to diagnosis and management*. Wiley, Chichester, pp. 303–18.

Jovanic-Peterson L, Peterson CM, Reed GF (1991). Maternal post-prandial glucose levels and infant birthweight: the Diabetes in Early Pregnancy Study. *Am J Obtet Gynecol* **164**: 103–11.

Lauenborg J, Mathiesen E, Ovesen P, Exbom P (2003). Audit on stillbirths in women with pregestational type 1 diabetes. *Diabetes Care* **26**: 1385–9.

Lepercq J, Taupin P, Dubois-Laforgue D (2001). Heterogeneity of fetal growth in type 1 diabetic pregnancy. *Diabetes Metab* **27**: 339–44.

Miller E, Hare JW, Clherty JP, Dunn PJ, Gleason RE (1981). Elevated maternal haemoglobinA1c in early pregnancy and major congenital anomolies in infants of diabetic mothers. *N Engl J Med* **304**: 1331-4.

Mimouni F, Tsang RC, Hertzberg VS, Miodovnik M (1986). Polycythemia, hypomagnesemia and hypocalcemia in infants of diabetic mothers. *Am J Dis Child* **140**: 798–800.

Peevy KJ, Lanaw SA, Gross SJ (1980). Hyperbilirubinemia in infants of diabetic mothers. *Pediatrics* **66**: 417–9.

Penney GC, Mair G, Pearson DWM (2003). Outcomes of pregnancies in women with type 1 diabetes in Scotland: a national population based study. *Br J Gynaecol* **110**: 315–8.

Pettitt DJ, Baird HR, Aleck KA, Bennett PH, Knowler WC (1983). Excessive obesity in offspring of Pima Indian women with diabetes during pregnancy. *N Engl J Med* **308**: 242–5.

Pettitt DJ, Aleck KA, Baird HR, Carraher MJ, Bennett PH, Knowler WC (1988). Congenital susceptibility to NIDDM. Role of intrauterine environment. *Diabetes* **37**: 622–8.

Reece EA, Pinter E, Homko C (1994). The yolk sac theory; closing the circle on why diabetes-associated malformations occur. *J Sco Gynecol Investig* **1**: 3–7.

Reece EA, Sivan E, Francis G, Homko CJ (1998). Pregnancy outcomes among women with and without diabetic microvascular disease versus non-diabetic controls. *Am J Perinatol* **15**: 549–55.

Robert MF, Neff RK, Hubbell JP (1976). Association between maternal diabetes and the respiratory-distress syndrome in the newborn. *N Engl J Med* **294**: 357–60.

Siddiqui F, James D (2003). Fetal monitoring in type 1 diabetic pregnancies. *Early Hum Dev* **72**: 1–13.

Sobgnwi E, Boudou P, Mauvais-Jarvis F, Leblanc H (2003). Effect of a diabetic environment in utero on predisposition to type 2 diabetes. *Lancet* **361**: 1861–5.

Stott A, Nik H, Platt MJ, Casson IF, Walkinshaw SA, Howard V (2004). Glycaemic control in pregnant women with type 1 diabetes and macrosomia. *Pract Diabetes Int* **21**: 215–20.

Stride A, Shepherd M, Frayling TM, Bulman MP, Ellard S, Hattersley AT (2002). Intrauterine hyperglycemia is associated with an earlier diagnosis of diabetes in HNF-1alpha gene mutation carriers. *Diabetes Care* **25**: 2287–91.

Ullmo S, Vial Y, Di Bernardo S (2007). Pathologic ventricular hypertrophy in the offspring of diabetic mothers: a retrospective study. *Eur Heart J* **28**: 1319–25.

Vaarasmaki M, Pota A, Elliot P (2009). Adolescent manifestations of metabolic syndrome among children born to women with gestational diabetes in a general population birth cohort. *Am J Epidemiol* **169**: 1209–15.

Way GL, Wolfe RR, Eshaghpour E (1979). The natural history of hypertrophic cardiomyopthy in infants of diabetic mothers. *J Pediatr* **95**: 1020-6.

Wren C, Birrell G, Hawthorne G (2003). Cardiovascular malformations in infants of diabetic mothers. *Heart* **89**: 1217–20.

Ylinen K, Aula P, Stenman U, Teramo K (1984). Risks of minor and major fetal malformations in diabetics with high haemoglobin HbA_{1c} values in early pregnancy. *Br Med J* **289**: 345–6.

Chapter 8

Postpartum management of women with diabetes

Rosemary Temple

Key points

- Insulin resistance drops immediately following delivery. There must be a clear management plan for glycaemic control following the birth
- Women should be supported to breastfeed
- Women with gestational diabetes are at high risk of developing diabetes or glucose intolerance in later life. They should have a glucose assessment six weeks following delivery and then annually
- Women with gestational diabetes should be educated about diet and lifestyle to reduce the risk of developing diabetes
- Education and advice about effective contraception should be given to all women with diabetes.

8.1 Diabetes management following birth

Immediately following the birth of the baby, insulin resistance falls dramatically. This should be anticipated, with a clear management plan to achieve good glycaemic control while avoiding hypoglycaemia. In women with type 1 diabetes (T1DM), insulin doses should be dropped to 70–80% of the pre-pregnancy insulin requirement. In addition, one needs to anticipate falls in glucose overnight due to glucose passing into breast milk. Management plans for women with pregestational and gestational diabetes are shown in Figures 8.1 and 8.2.

8.2 Breastfeeding in women with diabetes

The benefits of breastfeeding are well established and women with diabetes (DM) should be given education before delivery and

Fig 8.1 Postpartum management of women with gestational diabetes

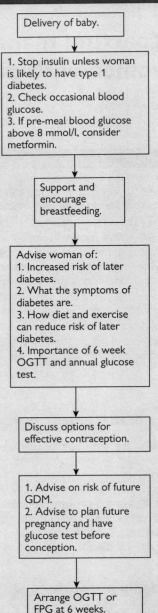

Delivery of baby.

1. Stop insulin unless woman is likely to have type 1 diabetes.
2. Check occasional blood glucose.
3. If pre-meal blood glucose above 8 mmol/l, consider metformin.

Support and encourage breastfeeding.

Advise woman of:
1. Increased risk of later diabetes.
2. What the symptoms of diabetes are.
3. How diet and exercise can reduce risk of later diabetes.
4. Importance of 6 week OGTT and annual glucose test.

Discuss options for effective contraception.

1. Advise on risk of future GDM.
2. Advise to plan future pregnancy and have glucose test before conception.

Arrange OGTT or FPG at 6 weeks.

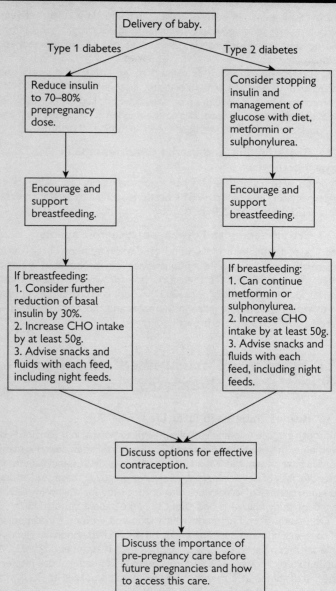

Fig 8.2 **Postpartum management of women with pregestational diabetes (type 1 and 2)**

Delivery of baby.

Type 1 diabetes   Type 2 diabetes

Reduce insulin to 70–80% prepregnancy dose.

Consider stopping insulin and management of glucose with diet, metformin or sulphonylurea.

Encourage and support breastfeeding.

Encourage and support breastfeeding.

If breastfeeding:
1. Consider further reduction of basal insulin by 30%.
2. Increase CHO intake by at least 50g.
3. Advise snacks and fluids with each feed, including night feeds.

If breastfeeding:
1. Can continue metformin or sulphonylurea.
2. Increase CHO intake by at least 50g.
3. Advise snacks and fluids with each feed, including night feeds.

Discuss options for effective contraception.

Discuss the importance of pre-pregnancy care before future pregnancies and how to access this care.

support following the birth to facilitate breastfeeding. Breastfeeding in women with T1DM is associated with a reduced risk of childhood obesity (OR, 0.3) (Humnel et al., 2009).

Establishing early feeding is paramount and time lapse between birth and first feeding should be minimized. Good glucose control during labour and delivery is essential to reduce risk of neonatal hypoglycaemia.

In T1DM, breastfeeding is related to gestation at delivery and infant birth weight rather than diabetes factors (Stage et al., 2006).

Women who are breastfeeding should be advised to increase carbohydrate intake by at least 50 g to reduce risk of hypoglycaemia and to snack and drink fluid with each feed, including all night feeds.

8.2.1 **Breastfeeding and insulin requirements in type 1 diabetes**

Women with T1DM need a reduction in insulin requirements of approximately 30%, which will be predominantly a reduction in basal insulin (Riviello et al., 2009).

8.2.2 **Breastfeeding and oral hypoglycaemic agents**

Studies of metformin and second-generation sulphonylureas have shown that only negligible amounts pass into breast milk with no effect on the infant. It is therefore safe for women taking these agents to breastfeed (Feig et al., 2007). There is no research into use of thiazolidinediones or incretin therapies and these are contraindicated in women who are breastfeeding.

8.3 **Postpartum management of women with gestational diabetes**

8.3.1 **Risk of diabetes in later life**

Although glucose tolerance usually returns to normal in the majority of women with gestational diabetes (GDM) shortly after delivery, many studies have shown there is an increased risk of developing diabetes in later life. Risk of developing diabetes varies greatly in these studies due to heterogeneity of factors including criteria used for diagnosing GDM, length of study follow-up and ethnicity of the patient population.

One study from Denmark, which followed women for a median of six years, showed 34.4% women with GDM had abnormal glucose tolerance compared to 5.3% control women (Damm et al., 1992). A further study showed 32.8% women with GDM had glucose intolerance or diabetes at 3 months after delivery compared to 3.2% in a control group (Retnakaran et al., 2008).

The Diabetes Prevention Programme Group has shown that a history of GDM in women with impaired glucose tolerance (IGT) further increases the risk of diabetes with an incidence rate of diabetes 71% higher in 350 women with IGT and previous GDM compared to 1,416 women with IGT and no previous GDM (Ratner et al., 2008).

Despite this high risk of later diabetes, recent studies suggest only 50% women have any glucose test in the first year following birth (Ferrara et al., 2009; Kwong et al., 2009).

One study of women with GDM reported that although 90% women recognized GDM as a risk factor for diabetes only 16% believed that they themselves were at risk of developing diabetes (Kim et al., 2007). This emphasises how important it is to educate women with GDM about their greatly increased risk of developing diabetes, including the symptoms of diabetes to enable early diagnosis and how to reduce risk of later diabetes.

8.3.2 Which test for diagnosis of diabetes following pregnancy?

NICE guidelines recommend measurement of fasting plasma glucose at 6 weeks and then annually to exclude glucose intolerance or diabetes (NICE, 2008). However, studies have shown measurement of fasting plasma glucose (FPG) alone rather than an oral glucose tolerance test (OGTT) would miss 38% to 72% of cases of glucose intolerance in women with GDM (Ferrara et al., 2009; Kwong et al., 2009). A recent systematic review of ten studies of postpartum screening tests in women with GDM which compared FPG with OGTT found that sensitivity ranged from 14% to 100% suggesting FPG is not a sensitive screening test (Bennett et al., 2009).

8.3.3 Risk factors for developing diabetes in later life

Studies of risk factors for later diabetes in women with GDM have often shown varied results. However, there are common features that healthcare professionals can use to identify those women at highest risk (Table 8.1). One study showed that FPG during pregnancy was the best predictor of later diabetes with 36.7% women developing diabetes if fasting glucose during pregnancy was above 6.7 mmol/l compared to only 0.5% women if fasting glucose was below 5.2 mmol/l (Schaefer-Graf et al., 2002).

8.4 Reducing the risk of later diabetes

8.4.1 Lifestyle

Both lifestyle intervention and metformin can successfully reduce the risk of developing diabetes in those at highest risk (Diabetes Prevention Programme (DPP) Research Group, 2002; Tuomilheto et al., 2001). Therefore, women with GDM should be encouraged to lose weight and take 150 minutes physical activity each week.

Table 8.1 Risk factors for development of diabetes in later life in women with gestational diabetes

Antepartum factors	Postpartum factors
High fasting glucose	High fasting glucose on postpartum OGTT
High glucose post-carbohydrate	High glucose at 2 hours on postpartum OGTT
Early gestational age at diagnosis of GDM	Increasing maternal age
High maternal BMI at booking	Maternal weight gain following pregnancy
Previous history of GDM	Additional pregnancy
Insulin treatment during pregnancy	
Low insulin secretion during OGTT	

Results of the DPP study showed women with GDM were less efficient at incorporating lifestyle changes compared to women without GDM, with less weight loss (1.6 kgs vs 4.03 kgs) and less physical activity at 3 years. However, lifestyle intervention still reduced risk of diabetes by 50% in GDM women (Ratner, 2008).

Women should be encouraged to have a diet low in high glycaemic carbohydrates as this further reduces risk of diabetes (Salmeron et al., 1997).

8.4.2 **Pharmacolgical agents**

The DPP study showed metformin is more effective in reducing risk of diabetes in women with GDM than those without GDM with 50.4% reduction in risk of diabetes in 350 women with GDM compared to 14.4% in 1,416 women without GDM (Ratner et al., 2008).

The Troglitazone In Prevention Of Diabetes study (TRIPOD study) and Pioglitazone In Prevention Of Diabetes study (PIPOD study) showed thiazolidinediones reduce insulin resistance and preserve beta cell function leading to a reduced incidence of diabetes in Hispanic GDM women (Xiang et al., 2006).

With the epidemics of type 2 diabetes and gestational diabetes upon us, there is a need for more long term studies of pharmaceutical agents in women with GDM.

8.5 **Contraception and planning future pregnancies**

It is mandatory to advise women about the importance of planning any future pregnancies, explaining how good glycaemic control in early pregnancy, use of folic acid supplements, avoidance of potentially teratogenic agents and weight management will optimize outcome. Women with GDM should be advised to have a glucose assessment before conception.

Short-term studies of low-dose combined oral contraceptive agents in women with T1DM have shown them to have minimal effect on diabetic control, lipid metabolism, and cardiovascular risk factors (Peterson et al., 1995). However, in women without diabetes, risk of myocardial infarction is increased in women with cardiovascular risk factors (especially hypertension) and cerebral thromboembolism is increased if there are pre-existing risk factors for stroke. Therefore, low-dose combined oral contraceptive agents appear safe for women with pregestational and gestational diabetes who have no co-existing vascular disease. For women with vascular disease, progesterone-only contraception should be recommended.

There is no increase in risk of later diabetes with the use of combined oral contraceptive agents in GDM women (Kjos et al., 1998).

Depot forms of progesterone contraception have been associated with an increase in incidence of type 2 diabetes in Navajo women (who are ethnically at high risk of diabetes), an increase in fasting and post-carbohydrate glucose levels and increase in weight and should be avoided in women with type 2 diabetes or previous GDM (Liew et al., 1985; Kim et al., 2001).

The Mirena® IUD is an effective form of contraception. It releases progesterone locally, decreases menstrual bleeding and atrophies the uterine lining. This may be a desirable benefit for obese women with type 2 diabetes or previous GDM who may be parous, older and at increased risk of endometrial cancer.

Further reading

Bennett WL, Bolen S, Wilson LM, et al. (2009). Performance characteristics of postpartum screening tests for type 2 diabetes mellitus in women with a history of gestational diabetes mellitus: a systematic review. J Womens Health (Larchmt) **18**: 979–87.

Damm P, Kuhl P, Bertelsen A, et al. (1992). Predictive factors for the development of diabetes in women with previous gestational diabetes. Am J Obstet Gynecol **167**: 607–16.

Davies HA, Clark JD, Dalton KJ, et al. (1989). Insulin requirements of diabetic women who breastfeed. BMJ **298**: 1357–8.

Diabetes Prevention Programme Research Group (2002). Reduction in the incidence of type 2 diabetes with lifestyle intervention or metformin. N Engl J Med **346**: 393–403.

Ferrara A, Peng T, Kim C (2009). Trends in postpartum diabetes screening and subsequent diabetes and impaired fasting glucose among women with histories of gestational diabetes mellitus: A report from the Translating Research Into Action for Diabetes (TRIAD) study. Diabetes Care **32**: 269–74.

Feig DS, Briggs GG, Koren G (2007). Oral antidiabetic agents in pregnancy and lactation: a paradigm shift? *Ann Pharmacother* **41**: 1174–80.

Humnel S, Pfluger M, Kreichauf S, *et al.* (2009). Predictors of overweight during childhood in offspring of parents with type 1 diabetes. *Diabetes Care* **32**: 921–5.

Kim C, Seidel KW, Degier EA, *et al.* (2001). Diabetes and depot medroxy-progesterone in Navajo women. *Arch Intern Med* **1616**: 1766–71.

Kim C, McEwen LN, Piette JD, *et al.* (2007). Risk perception for diabetes among women with histories of gestational diabetes mellitus. *Diabetes Care* **30**: 2281–6.

Kjos SL, Shoupe D, Douyan S, *et al.* (1998). Contraception and the risk of type 2 diabetes mellitus in Latina women with prior gestational diabetes mellitus. *Am J Med Assoc* **280**: 533–8.

Kwong S, Mitchell RS, Senior PA, *et al.* (2009). Postpartum diabetes screening: adherence rate and the performance of fasting glucose versus oral glucose tolerance test. *Diabetes Care* **32**: 2242–4.

Liew DFM, Ng CS, Young YM, *et al.* (1985). Long-term effects of depo-provera on carbohydrate and lipid metabolism. *Contraception* **31**: 51–64.

Peterson KR, Skouby SO, Vedel P, *et al.* (1995). Hormonal contraception in women with IDDM. *Diabetes Care* **18**: 800–6.

Ratner RE, Christophi CA, Metzger BE, *et al.* (2008). Prevention of diabetes in women with a history of gestational diabetes: effects of metformin and lifestyle interventions. *J Clin Endocrinol Metab* **93**: 4774–9.

Retnakaran R, Qi Y, Sermer M, *et al.* (2008). Glucose intolerance in pregnancy and future risk of pre-diabetes or diabetes. *Diabetes Care* **31**: 2026–31.

Riviello C, Mello G, Jovanovic L (2009). Breastfeeding and the basal insulin requirement in type 1 diabetic women. *Endocr Pract* **15**: 187–93.

Salmeron J, Asherio A, Rimm EB, *et al.* (1997). Dietary fiber, glycaemic load and risk of NIDDM in men. *Diabetes Care* **20**: 545–50.

Schaefer-Graf UM, Buchanan TA, Xiang AH, *et al.* (2002). Clinical predictors for a high risk for the development of diabetes mellitus in the early puerperium in women with recent gestational diabetes mellitus. *Am J Obstet Gynecol* **186**: 751–6.

Stage E, Norgard H, Damm P, *et al.* (2006). Lonterm breastfeeding in women with type 1 diabetes. *Diabetes Care* **29**: 771–4.

Tuomilheto J, Lindstrom J, Eriksson JG *et al.* (2001). Prevention of type 2 diabetes by changes in lifestyle among subjects with impaired glucose tolerance. *N Engl J Med* **344**: 1343–50.

Xiang AH, Peters RK, Kjos SL, *et al.* (2006). Effect of pioglitazone on pancreatic betacell function and diabetes risk in Hispanic women with prior gestational diabetes. *Diabetes* **55**: 517–22.

Chapter 9

Drugs and breastfeeding in women with diabetes

Denice S Feig

Key points

- When prescribing drugs to a breastfeeding mother careful consideration of passage of drugs into breast milk and potential effects on the infant needs to be made
- Of the oral hypoglycaemics metformin appears to pass into breast milk in only tiny quantities and can be considered for use, although caution is advised while nursing premature infants and those with renal impairment. More limited evidence supports use of selected sulphonylureas (glibenclamide, glipizide)
- Antihypertensive agents commonly used in pregnancy (methyldopa, labetalol, nifedipine) can also be considered in breastfeeding mothers along with selected beta blockers and ACE inhibitors
- Breastfeeding exerts many benefits for the mother and child and should be encouraged. Recent evidence suggests that there may be long-term benefits reducing the risk of obesity and type 2 diabetes in offspring.

There are several circumstances in which women with diabetes may find that they need to take medications during lactation. Prior to pregnancy many women with type 2 diabetes take oral antihyperglycaemic agents for glycaemic control. These oral agents are usually discontinued in pregnancy and replaced by insulin. Once the baby is born, however, many women prefer to switch back to pills because of their ease of administration and low cost. Women with diabetes often have chronic hypertension and require antihypertensive therapy during the period of lactation. They may also have underlying nephropathy and require renal protection. As well, physicians may wish to use metformin during breastfeeding in women with a history of gestational diabetes, as studies have demonstrated that metformin is effective in delaying or preventing diabetes in women with a history of gestational diabetes (Ratner et al., 2008). In this chapter we will review whether these drugs needed for glycaemic control, blood pressure control, and renal protection, pass into breastmilk, and whether they are considered safe during breastfeeding (see also Table 9.1). We will also review some potential long-term benefits of breastfeeding in offspring of women with diabetes.

9.1 **Oral antihyperglycemic agents and breastfeeding**

9.1.1 **Metformin**

Metformin is a biguanide and, after diet and exercise, is often recommended as the first line of drug therapy for the treatment of type 2 diabetes. It acts by reducing hepatic gluconeogenesis, increasing peripheral glucose uptake in skeletal muscle and adipocytes, and by reducing intestinal glucose absorption (Hundal et al., 2000; Cusi & DeFronzo, 1998). There are several advantages to the use of metformin. Metformin does not cause weight gain, nor does it cause hypoglycemia (Kirpichnikov et al., 2002). Metformin has also been shown to decrease progression to type 2 diabetes in women with gestational diabetes (Ratner et al., 2008), and it has been shown to improve ovulatory rates in women with polycystic ovary syndrome (Lord et al., 2003).

To date there have been three studies published looking at the transfer of metformin into breastmilk (Hale et al., 2002; Briggs et al., 2005; Gardiner et al., 2003). In these studies, women were either taking 500 mg BID-TID, 500 mg per day in a slow release form, or a single dose of 500 mg. Metformin was detected in the breastmilk, with the mean milk to plasma ratios calculated in these studies ranging from 0.35 to 0.63. The estimated infant dose normalized for the mother's weight-adjusted dose was 0.11% to 0.65%, meaning the infant received only 0.65% of the mother's weight-adjusted dose. This is well below the theoretically acceptable level of 10% (Hale et al., 2002; Bennett, 1996). Blood samples for metformin were taken in six infants. Metformin was either undetectable (in four) or found at very low concentration (in two). All nursing infants were found to be healthy, and two infants tested using the Denver Developmental Screening test were normal for age (Hale et al., 2002). Glucose levels tested in 2 infants were also normal (2.6 to 4.3 mmol/l) (Briggs et al., 2005).

In a longer-term study, 61 nursing infants were compared to 50 formula-fed infants of mothers taking metformin (median dose

Table 9.1 Compatibility of drugs with breastfeeding

	Compatible with breastfeeding	Not compatible with breastfeeding
Oral antihyperglycaemic agents		
Metformin	√[a]	
Glibenclamide	√[b]	
Glipizide	√[b]	
Thiazolidinediones		No information
DPP IV inhibitors		No information
GLP-1 agonists		No information
Antihypertensives		
Methyldopa	√	
Labetalol	√	
Nifedipine	√	
Beta-blockers		
Atenolol		Not recommended
Acebutolol		Not recommended
Metoprolol	√	
Propranolol	√	
Oxyprenolol	√	
Nadolol		Not first line
Sotalol		Not first line
ACE inhibitors		
Captopril[c]	√	
Enalopril[c]	√	
Quinapril[c]	√	
Angiotensin II receptor blockers		No information

[a] While metformin appears to be compatible with breastfeeding, caution is advised while nursing premature infants and those with renal impairment.

[b] While glibenclamide and glipizide appear compatible with breastfeeding, until more data are available, it may be prudent to watch for hypoglycemia or monitor glucose levels in the baby.

[c] Note that the *British National Formulary* suggests that 'Captopril, enalapril, and quinapril should be avoided in the first few weeks after delivery, particularly in preterm infants, due to the risk of profound neonatal hypotension; if essential, they may be used in mothers breast-feeding older infants—the infant's blood pressure should be monitored.'

2.5 g per day) throughout pregnancy and lactation, for polycystic ovary syndrome (Glueck *et al.*, 2004). At 6 months of age, weight, height, and motor-social development did not differ between the groups. None of the infants had a delay in growth, motor or social development. While metformin appears to be compatible with breastfeeding, caution is advised while nursing premature infants and those with renal impairment.

9.1.2 **Sulphonylureas**

Sulphonylureas act by increasing insulin secretion. The first-generation sulphonylureas, tolbutamide and chlorpropamide, have been shown to cross into breast milk (Moiel & Ryan, 1967; Everett, 1997). To date only one study has examined the transfer of second-generation sulphonylureas, glibenclamide (glyburide) and glipizide, into breastmilk (Feig *et al.*, 2005). Women received either a single dose of glibenclamide (5 or 10 mg), or given a daily dosage of 5 mg/day of glyburide or glipizide. Neither glibenclamide nor glipizide were detected in any of the milk samples. Blood glucose levels were normal in the three nursing infants tested. While glibenclamide and glipizide are likely safe, because of the paucity of data available, it is prudent to monitor glucose levels in the baby.

9.1.3 **Thiazolidenediones, DPP IV inhibitors, GLP-1 agonists**

To date there is no information regarding the transfer into breastmilk or safety of thiazolidenediones, DPP IV inhibitors, or GLP-1 agonists during lactation in humans. Their use during lactation is not recommended.

9.2 **Antihypertensives/renal protection and breastfeeding**

Women with diabetes have an increased risk of chronic hypertension and pre-eclampsia. Therefore, a number of women will require antihypertensive medication during lactation.

Methyldopa, labetalol and nifedipine are considered the preferred agents for use in pregnancy (Powrie, 2007). Low levels of these agents are found in breast milk (Jones & Cummings, 1978; White *et al.*, 1985; Hauser *et al.*, 1985; Ehrenkranz *et al.*, 1989; Taddio *et al.*, 1996; Leitz *et al.*, 1983; Lunell *et al.*, 1985; Atkinson *et al.*, 1988) and all are considered compatible with breastfeeding (Bennett, 1996; Committee, 2001).

The excretion of beta-blockers into breastmilk varies widely depending on their plasma protein binding. Atenolol and acebutolol are found in high levels in breastmilk (Beardmore *et al.*, 2002), and because of reports of adverse effects in exposed infants (Schmimmel et al., 1989; Boutroy et al., 1986), they are not recommended in nursing infants (Committee, 2001). Metoprolol, propranolol and oxprenolol, are considered compatible with breastfeeding, whereas nadolol and sotalol are found in high levels in breastmilk, and are not considered first-line agents in breastfeeding mothers (Briggs et al., 2005, Hale 2006).

The use of angiotensin-converting enzyme inhibitors and angiotensin II receptor blockers is contraindicated during pregnancy, however, several women with diabetes, especially those with diabetic nephropathy, may want to use these agents postpartum for control of hypertension and renal protection. Captopril, enalapril and quinapril are found in low levels in breastmilk, and no adverse effects have been reported in breastfed infants (Hutunen et al., 1989; Rush et al., 1991; Redman et al., 1990; Begg et al., 2001). There are no reports to date examining the use of the angiotensin II receptor blockers during lactation.

9.3 Breastfeeding and long-term benefits to women and their infants of women with diabetes

While the short-term benefits of breastfeeding are well known, there are increasing data to suggest breastfeeding confers some positive long-term benefits to infants of women with diabetes.

9.3.1 Benefits to offspring

9.3.1.1 Obesity

Breastfeeding has been shown to decrease the risk of obesity in infants of non-diabetic mothers by 13–22% in two meta-analyses (Arenz et al., 2004; Owen et al., 2005). Another meta-analysis confirmed the association to be dose-dependent, with longer duration of breastfeeding leading to a decreased risk of overweight later in life (Harder et al., 2005). It is hypothesized that over-nutrition from bottle-feeding, in the early postnatal period, may lead to accelerated early neonatal growth, which has been associated with overweight in childhood and adulthood (Stettler et al., 2002). In children of mothers with diabetes, however, the evidence is somewhat conflicting. Studies looking at overweight in children aged 1–2 years, showed either an increase in risk of overweight in mothers who breastfed compared to those given donor (non-diabetic) breastmilk (Plagemann et al., 2002), or no association (Kerrsen et al., 2004) in women with diabetes who breastfed. Studies looking at older children, however, were more positive. In the Nurses Health Study, children of women with diabetes who were exclusively breastfed, had a reduced risk of overweight at age 9–14 years (Mayer-Davis et al., 2006). More recent studies in women with gestational diabetes (Schaeffer-Graf et al., 2006) and women with type 1 diabetes (Hummel et al., 2009), found significant reductions in childhood overweight in children aged 5–8 years who were breastfed more than 3–4 months.

9.3.1.2 Diabetes

Studies in offspring of non-diabetic women show a reduced risk of type 2 diabetes with breastfeeding. In a meta-analysis of 23 studies, breastfeeding reduced the risk of type 2 diabetes by 39% (Owen et al., 2006). In a recent case-control study of 80 youths with type 2 diabetes compared to normal controls, breastfeeding was protective against type 2 diabetes (Mayer-Davis et al., 2008).

Studies in women with type 1 diabetes suggest that breastfeeding may decrease the risk of type 1 diabetes in genetically susceptible offspring (Virtanen et al., 2003). It is hypothesized that cow's milk protein may trigger an autoimmune response. A randomized trial comparing casein hydrolysate with a conventional cow's milk-based formula in children at increased risk of type 1 diabetes is currently underway to answer this question (The TRIGR Study Group).

There are no data in offspring of women with type 2 diabetes and their risk of type 2 diabetes following breastfeeding, however, breastfeeding lowered the risk of type 2 diabetes in children of Pima Indian women who have a very high risk of type 2 diabetes (Pettit et al., 1997).

9.3.2 **Benefits to women**

There is increasing evidence that breastfeeding is beneficial to women as well as their offspring. Two large prospective studies looking at over 80,000 non-diabetic women in the Nurses' Health Study found that longer duration of breastfeeding was associated with reduced rates of type 2 diabetes (Stuebe et al., 2005) and coronary heart disease (Stuebe et al., 2009). In another prospective study of 139,681 postmenopausal non-diabetic women in the Women's Health Initiative, increased duration of lactation was associated with lowered rates of hypertension, diabetes, hyperlipidemia and cardiovascular disease (Schwarz et al., 2009). Women with gestational diabetes may also benefit. In a recent study of 1,399 women in the Coronary Artery Risk Development in Young Adults (CARDIA) study, longer duration of lactation was associated with lower incidence of metabolic syndrome in women with and without a history of gestational diabetes (Gunderson et al., 2010). To date there are no data on lactation and the risk of hypertension or cardiovascular disease in women with type 1 or type 2 diabetes.

Further reading

Arenz S, Ruckerl R, Koletzko B, von Kries R (2004). Breast-feeding and childhood obesity: a systematic review. *Int J Obes Relat* **28**: 1247–56.

Atkinson HC, Begg EJ, Darlow BA (1998). Drugs in human milk. Clinical pharmacokinetic considerations. *Clin Pharmacokinet* **14**: 217–40.

Beardmore KS, Morris JM, Gallery EDM (2002). Excretion of antihypertensive medication into human breast milk: A systematic review. *Hypertension in Pregnancy* **21**: 85–95.

Begg EJ, Robson RA, Gardiner SJ, et al. (2001). Quinapril and its metabolite quinaprilat in human milk. *J Clin Pharmacol* **51**: 478–81.

Bennett PN (1996). *Drugs and Human Lactation*, 2nd edition. Elsevier Science, London.

Boutroy MJ, Bianchetti G, Dubruc C, Vert P, Morselli PL (1986). To nurse when receiving acebutolol: is it dangerous for the neonate? *Eur J Clin Pharmacol* **30**: 737–9.

Briggs GG, Ambrose PJ, Nageotte MP, et al. (2005). Excretion of metformin into breast milk and the effect on nursing infants. *Obstet Gynecol* **105**: 1437–41.

Briggs GG, Freeman RK, Yaffe SJ (2005). *Drugs in Pregnancy and Lactation: A Reference Guide to Fetal And Neonatal Risk.* Lippincott Williams & Wilkins, Philadelphia, PA, USA.

Committee on Drugs, American Academy of Pediatrics (2001). The transfer of drugs and other chemicals into human milk. *Pediatrics* **108**: 776–89.

Cusi K, DeFronzo RA (1998). Metformin: a review of its metabolic effects. *Diabetes Review* **6**: 89–131.

Ehrenkranz RA, Ackerman BA, Hulse JD (1989). Nifedipine transfer into human milk. *J Pediatr* **114**: 478–80.

Everett JA (1997). Use of oral antidiabetic agents during breastfeeding. *J Hum Lact* **13**: 319–21.

Feig DS, Briggs GG, Kraemer JM, et al. (2005). Transfer of glyburide and glipizide into breast milk. *Diabetes Care* **28**: 1851–5.

Gardiner SJ, Kirkpatrick CM, Begg EJ, et al. (2003). Transfer of metformin into human milk. *Clin Pharmacol Ther* **73**: 71–7.

Glueck CJ, Godenberg N, Pranikoff J, et al. (2004). Height, weight and motor-social development during the first 18 months of life in 126 infants born to 109 mothers with polycystic ovary syndrome who conceived on and continued metformin through pregnancy. *Human Reproduction* **19**: 1323–30.

Gunderson EP, Jacobs DR, Chiang V, et al. (2010). Duration of lactation and incidence of the metabolic syndrome in women of reproductive age according to gestational diabetes mellitus status: A 20-year prospective study in CARDIA (Coronary Artery Risk Development in Young Adults). *Diabetes* **59**: 495–504.

Hale TW, Kristensen JH, Hackett LP, et al. (2002). Transfer of metformin into human milk. *Diabetologia* **45**: 1509–1514.

Harder T, Bergmann R, Kallischinigg G, Plagemann A (2005). Duration of breastfeeding and risk of overweight: a meta-analysis. *Am J Epidemiol* **162**: 397–403.

Hauser GJ, Almog S, Tirosh M, *et al.* (1985). Effect of alpha-methyl-dopa excreted in human milk on the breast-fed infant. *Helv Paediatr Acta* **40**: 83–6.

Ho TK, Moretti ME, Schaeffer JK, *et al.* (1999). Maternal beta-blocker usage and breast feeding in the neonate. *Pediatr Res* **45**: 67A, abstract 385.

Hummel S, Pfluger M, Kreichauf S, Hummel M, Ziegler A (2009). Predictors of overweight during childhood in offspring of parents with type 1 diabetes. *Diabetes Care* **32**: 921–5.

Hundal RS, Krssak M, Dufours S, *et al.* (2000). Mechanism by which metformin reduces glucose production in type 2 diabetes. *Diabetes* **49**: 2063–9.

Huttunen K, Gronhagen-Riska C, Fyhrquist F (1989). Enalpril treatment of a nursing mother with slightly impaired renal function. *Clin Nephrol* **31**: 278.

Jones HMR, Cummings AJ (1978). A study of the transfer of alpha-methyldopa to the human foetus and newborn infant. *Br J Clin Pharmacol* **6**: 432–4.

Kerssen A, Evers IM, de Valk HW, Visser GHA (2004). Effect of breast milk of diabetic mothers on bodyweight of the offspring in the first year of life. *European Journal of Clinicl Nutrition* **58**: 1429–31.

Kirpichnikov D, McFarlane SI, Sowers JR (2002). Metformin: an update. *Ann Intern Med* **137**: 25–33.

Leitz F, Bariletto S, Gural R, *et al.* (1983). Secretion of labetalol in breast milk of lactatin women. *Fed Proc* **42**: 378, abstract.

Lord J, Flight I, Normal R (2003). Insulin-sensitising drugs (metformin, troglitazone, rosiglitazone, pioglitazone, D-chiro-inositol) for polycystic ovary syndrome. *Cochrane Database Syst Rev* Issue: CD003053.

Lunell NO, Kulas J, Rane A (1985). Transfer of labetalol into amniotic fluid and breast milk in lactating women. *Eur J Clin Pharmacol* **28**: 597–9.

Mayer-Davis EJ, Rifas-Shiman SL, Zhou L, Hu FB, Colditz GA, Gillman MW (2006). Breast-feeding and risk for childhood obesity; Does maternal diabetes or obesity status matter? *Diabetes Care* **29**: 2231–7.

Mayer-Davis EJ, Dabelea D, Lamichhane AP, *et al.* (2008). Breast-feeding and type 2 diabetes in the youth of three ethnic groups: the SEARCH for diabetes in youth case-control study. *Diabetes Care* Mar **31**: 470–5.

Moiel RH, Ryan JR (1967). Tolbutamide orinase in human breast milk. *Clinical Ped* **6**: 480.

Owen CG, Martin RM, Whincup PH, Smith GD, Cook DG (2005). Effect of infant feeding on the risk of obesity across the life course: a quantitative review of published evidence. *Pediatrics* **15**: 1367–77.

Owen CG, Martin RM, Whincup PH, Davey Smith G, Cook DG (2006). Does breastfeeding influence risk of type 2 diabetes in later life? A quantitative analysis of published evidence. *Am J Clin Nutr* **84**: 1043–54.

Pettitt DJ, Forman MR, Hanson RL, Knowler WC, Bennett PH (1997). Breastfeeding and incidence of non-insulin-dependent diabetes mellitus in Pima Indians. *Lancet* **350**: 166–8.

Plagemann A, Harder T, Franke K, Kohlhoff R (2002). Long-term impact of neonatal breastfeeding on body weight and glucose tolerance in children of diabetic mothers. *Diabetes Care* **25**: 16–22.

Powrie RO (2007). A 30 year old woman with chronic hypertension trying to conceive. *JAMA* **298**: 1548–58.

Ratner RE, Christophi CA, Metzger BE, et al., and The Diabetes Prevention Program Research Group (2008). Prevention of diabetes in women with a history of gestational diabetes: effects of metformin and lifestyle interventions. *J Clin Endocrinol Metab* **93**: 4774–9.

Redman CWG, Kelly JG, Cooper WD (1990). The excretion of enalapril and enalaprilat in human breast milk. *Eur J Clin Pharmacol* **38**: 99.

Rush JE, Snyder DL, Barrish A, et al. (1991). Comment on Huttunen K, Gronhagen-Riska C, Fyhrquist F. Enalpril treatment of a nursing mother with slightly impaired renal function. *Clin Nephrol* **35**: 234 (letter).

Sandstrom B, Regardh CG (1980). Metoprolol excretion into breast milk. *Br J Clin Pharmacol* **9**: 518–9.

Schaeffer-Graf UM, Hartmann R, Pawliczak J, et al. (2006). Association of breast-feeding and early childhood overweight in children from mothers with gestational diabetes mellitus. *Diabetes Care* **29**: 1105–7.

Schmimmel MS, Eidelman AJ, Wilschanski MA, Shaw D Jr, Ogilvie RJ, Koren G (1989). Toxic effects of atenolol consumed during breastfeeding. *J Pediatr* **114**: 476–8.

Schwarz EB, Ray RM, Stuebe B, et al. (2009). Duration of lactation and risk factors for maternal cardiovascular disease. *Obstet Gynecol* **113**: 974–82.

Stettler N, Zemel BS, Kumanyika S, Stallings VA (2002). Infant weight gain and childhood overweight status in a multicenter, cohort study. *Pediatrics* **109**: 194–9.

Stuebe AM, Rich-Edwards JW, Willett WC, Manson J, Michels KB (2005). Duration of lactation and incidence of type 2 diabetes. *JAMA* 2601–10.

Stuebe AM, Michels KB, Willett WC, Manson JE, Rexrode K, Rich-Edwards JW (2009). Duration of lactation and incidence of myocardial infarction in middle to late adulthood. *Am J Obstet Gynecol* **200**: 138.e1–138.e8.

Taddio A, Oskamp M, Ito S, et al. (1996). Is nifedipine use during labour and breastfeeding safe for the neonate? *Clin Invest Med* **19**: S11, abstract.

Virtanen SM, Knip M (2003). Nutritinal rsk predictors of beta cell autoimmunity and type 1 diabetes at a young age. *Am J Clin Nutr* **78**: 1053–67.

White WB, Andreoli JW, Wong SH, Cohn RD (1984). Atenolol in human plasma and breast milk. *Obstet Gynecol* **63**: 42S–44S.

White WB, Andreoli JW, Cohn RD (1985). Alpha-methyldopa disposition in mothers with hypertension and in their breast-fed infants. *Clin Pharmacol Ther* **37**: 387–90.

Index

Page numbers in *italic* indicate figures and tables.

Diet

Only to have 30g of carbs per meal.

→ what effects blood glucose readings.

→ sugar carbs, starchy carbs hidden sugars - milk and fruit.

glucose for energy.

insulin → glucose to energy in the body.

reduce carbs.

→ what protein do they like in diet.

→ fruit - high glucose, salad, veg.

| berries | | nuts |

→ cauliflower rice

vaccines elearning
time back for that!

Dating scan -
HbA1c and Random
HBA1c ↑ 41
random ↑ 9 mmols.

* Antenatal care -

- pre-existing diabetes and high
  BGLS - increased risk of abnormal
  stillbirth and miscarriage.
- Babies need glucose to grow

- 20 weeks, placental hormones
  cause insulin resistance in the
  mothers cells.

- Insulin resistant cells are less
  able to convert glucose into
  energy, resulting in a peak of
  blood glucose which goes through
  the placenta to 'feed' the baby.

- 4 x daily min blood sugar
  levels.

→ fasting and one hour after each
  meal.
→ treatment important.

Aim - 3.5 - 7.8.

metformin - renal function
normal.

- All appointments - meter and
  blood glucose diary.

* Care in Labour -

- Increased risk of shoulder dystocia, perineal tearing.

- Insulin can also delay the production of surfactant, which prepares the lungs for breathing

- two increased risks of neonatal hypoglycaemia poorly controlled BSLs in late pregnancy + maternal hyperglycaemia during labour.

✱ Postnatal care –

- Primary visit
- ? BST
  and discharge visit.

- GP to follow up GDM @ ▬▬▬
  postnatal.

✱ Jaundice – baby's high insulin
  levels during pregnancy increase
  their red blood cells.